The Profession of Dietetics

SIXTH EDITION

A TEAM APPROACH

June R. Payne-Palacio, PhD
Professor Emeritus
Pepperdine University

Deborah D. Canter, PhD, RD, LD, FAND
Professor Emeritus
Kansas State University

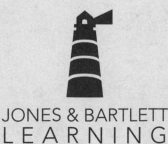

JONES & BARTLETT
LEARNING

World Headquarters
Jones & Bartlett Learning
5 Wall Street
Burlington, MA 01803
978-443-5000
info@jblearning.com
www.jblearning.com

Jones & Bartlett Learning books and products are available through most bookstores and online booksellers. To contact Jones & Bartlett Learning directly, call 800-832-0034, fax 978-443-8000, or visit our website, www.jblearning.com.

Substantial discounts on bulk quantities of Jones & Bartlett Learning publications are available to corporations, professional associations, and other qualified organizations. For details and specific discount information, contact the special sales department at Jones & Bartlett Learning via the above contact information or send an email to specialsales@jblearning.com.

Production Credits

VP, Executive Publisher: David D. Cella
Publisher: Cathy L. Esperti
Acquisitions Editor: Sean Fabery
Vendor Manager: Sara Kelly
Director of Marketing: Andrea DeFronzo
VP, Manufacturing and Inventory Control: Therese Connell
Composition and Project Management: Cenveo Publisher Services
Cover Design: Kristin E. Parker
Rights & Media Specialist: Jamey O'Quinn
Media Development Editor: Troy Liston
Cover Image: © XiXinXing/Shutterstock
Printing and Binding: Edwards Brothers Malloy
Cover Printing: Edwards Brothers Malloy

Library of Congress Cataloging-in-Publication Data
Names: Payne-Palacio, June, author. | Canter, Deborah D., author.
Title: The profession of dietetics : a team approach / June R. Payne-Palacio, Deborah D. Canter.
Description: 6th edition. | Burlington, MA : Jones & Bartlett Learning, [2017] | Includes bibliographical references and index.
Identifiers: LCCN 2016018645 | ISBN 9781284101850 (pbk. : alk. paper)
Subjects: | MESH: Dietetics | Patient Care Team | Vocational Guidance | United States
Classification: LCC RM218.5 | NLM WB 400 | DDC 613.2023—dc23
LC record available at https://lccn.loc.gov/2016018645

6048

Printed in the United States of America
20 19 18 17 16   10 9 8 7 6 5 4 3 2

B R I E F

C O N T E N T S

CONTENTS

The Profession of Dietetics: A Team Approach is written for students interested in finding out more about the profession of dietetics. Understanding who dietetics professionals are, what dietetics professionals do, and how to become a certified dietary manager; a nutrition and dietetics technician, registered; or a registered dietitian nutritionist is a complex task. Few other professions offer so many educational routes for entry or so many ways to practice one's trade. While this diversity is a strength, it often confuses those who wish to enter the profession, as well as prospective customers who are trying to understand who dietetics professionals are or why they should consult one.

It is the goal of this book to present a clear and up-to-date picture of the profession of dietetics and to try to answer some basic questions:

- What is a profession and how does dietetics qualify as a profession?
- How has the history of the profession shaped dietetics practice today?
- Who are members of the dietetics team and how do they work together?
- What is the Academy of Nutrition and Dietetics (formerly the American Dietetic Association) and why should one become a member?
- What is involved in the credentialing of dietetics professionals and why is it important?
- What kinds of positions do dietetics professionals fill?
- Why are communication and teamwork so important in the dietetics profession?
- How can a person develop effective communication skills and become a good team player?
- What are some ways to successfully make the transition from student to professional?
- What does the future hold for dietetics practice?

Features throughout the text are designed to help students connect with the material presented. Suggested Activities at the end of each chapter allow students to explore topics further and offer opportunities for thought-provoking research outside the classroom. Selected websites direct students to view related content online and to peruse a variety of Web pages pertaining to the field of dietetics. The ever-popular Profile of a Professional feature includes real interviews with individuals who work in various positions as dietetics professionals. Each professional who is profiled offers advice and words of wisdom for students entering the field.

Qualified instructors can also receive access to instructor resources including a test bank, slides in PowerPoint format, and an instructor's manual.

The profession of dietetics is dynamic, exciting, and in need of enthusiastic, energetic, and visionary men and women who wish to join the team. It is our hope that this book enlightens, informs, and inspires those who read it. If this occurs, then our dream for this book will have been achieved.

This edition of *The Profession of Dietetics: A Team Approach* reflects the latest standards, developments, and data in the dynamic and constantly evolving field of dietetics. Key changes for this edition include the following:

- Seventeen all-new *Profile of a Professional* features, spotlighting the experiences and accomplishments of both dietitians and dietetic technicians
- The latest numbers relating to the growth of the profession, including employment outlook, median salary expectations, and new program accreditation
- The highlighting of digital portfolios and the utility of LinkedIn and other digital career resources
- Updated information regarding education requirements, reflecting the most recent changes announced by the Academy of Nutrition and Dietetics

Major chapter-specific updates are listed below.

Part I: The Past

Chapter 1: The Profession Is Born

- Adds references to the recently introduced RDN and NDTR credential
- Updates timeline of selected milestones in dietetic history
- Includes discussion of Marjorie Hulsizer Copher's contributions during World War I

Part II: The Present

Chapter 2: The Dietetics Profession

- Updates the discussion surrounding the various titles and credentials a dietitian may use
- Features the latest statistics on
  - RDN and NDTR median salaries
  - Top-paying states and metropolitan areas for professionals
  - Projected growth in employment through 2022
- Integrates today's understanding of food's role in preventing and treating diseases
- Discusses the Academy's development of Board Certification in some specialty areas of dietetic practice

Chapter 3: Join Together: The Team Approach

- Incorporates current titles and credentials for all team members

Chapter 4: Beginning Your Path to Success in Dietetics

- Updates portfolio (now profile) information to emphasize digital career resources like LinkedIn and other social media platforms
- Adds a section on digital portfolios (e-portfolios)
- Incorporates new formatting and stylistic tips for résumés
- Adds and updates interviewing tips
- Supplies a variety of online resources for assistance with online self-marketing, job searching, e-portfolios, and interviews

Part III: Preparing for Practice

Chapter 5: Dietetics Education and Training

- Describes the two current options for becoming a dietetic technician
- Details ACEND's recommendation that the master's degree become the standard for all entry-level dietitians and the controversy surrounding this move
- Incorporates information regarding the differences in salaries between RDNs with a master's degree and those with a bachelor's degree

Chapter 6: The Supervised Practice Experience

- Addresses the dietetic internship shortage in a new section, providing the latest statistics and explanations for why the shortage is occurring
- Delves into reasons why students are increasingly taking more than 4 years to graduate with a bachelor's degree
- Provides more detail regarding distance internships and their admission criteria

Chapter 7: Credentialing

- Provides the latest statistics for the number of dietitians, dietetic technicians, and various specialty credentials
- Addresses the Academy's new Fellow of the Academy of Nutrition and Dietetics program
- Provides advisory information on researching and preparing for state licensure

Part IV: Professional Organizations

Chapter 8: Why Join a Professional Association?

- Updates the distinction between active members, retired members, and academy associates of the Academy of Nutrition and Dietetics
- Updates the presentation of the Academy's vision, mission, and values

- Adds the Academy's Governing Structure Infographic to outline the membership, functions, management responsibilities, and frequency of meetings for both the Board of Directors and the House of Delegates
- Updates the listing of Dietetic Practice Groups (DPGs) and Member Interest Groups (MIGs)
- Expands the list of awards and grants offered by the Academy
- Lists and describes affiliate award programs

Part V: The Future

Chapter 9: Trends, Predictions, and Your Future

- Describes the change drivers and trends for the dietetics profession that have been identified by the Council on Future Practice
- Delves into the implications of these change drivers and trends on dietetic practice

Chapter 10: Crossing the Bridge: From Student to Professional

- Distinguishes Standards of Practice (SOP) from Standards of Professional Performance (SOPP) and describes by whom and how they are used

ACKNOWLEDGMENTS

We owe a debt of gratitude to Karen Lechowich at the Academy of Nutrition and Dietetics who, because of her love of this profession and its history, went "above and beyond the call of duty" in her efforts to help us with this project. We would also like to express special thanks to our editorial and production staff at Jones & Bartlett Learning for their patience while working with us and for their support and encouragement for the completion of this revision, especially Sean Fabery, who pushed and prodded us at the right times, always with tact and diplomacy, to make sure this book was published on time. His guidance and wise suggestions made this a better book.

We wish to acknowledge the special people in our lives who helped us through the production of this edition. Appreciation is expressed to Deb's "adopted family," Rebecca and Jeff Daniels and children Hope (along with her husband Sam and new daughter Sophia), Ian, Grace, Nigel, and Gavin in Overland Park, Kansas. Many thanks also are expressed to friends Sharon and Medo Morcos in Manhattan, who share so much love and support. Special love and appreciation are also expressed to June's husband, Cliff Duboff, for his emotional support and untiring help. And, finally, we thank the dietetics students at Pepperdine University, Kansas State University, and across the country who daily confirm our belief in the secure future of the profession of dietetics.

REVIEWERS

Judith Anglin, PhD, RDN
Director of Dietetics
Associate Professor
Texas Southern University
Houston, TX

Carol Beier, MS, RD/LD
Director, Didactic Program in
    Dietetics
Oklahoma State University
Stillwater, OK

Elise Cowie, MEd, RD, LD
Director, Coordinated Program in
    Dietetics
Assistant Professor
University of Cincinnati
Cincinnati, OH

Amy A. Drescher, PhD, RD
Instructor
Central Arizona College
Coolidge, AZ

Andrea Hutchins, PhD, RD
Associate Professor
University of Colorado Springs
Colorado Springs, CO

Dorothy Chen Maynard, PhD, RD,
    FAND
Director, Directed Program in
    Dietetics
Associate Professor
California State University, San
    Bernardino
San Bernardino, CA

Lisa Sheehan-Smith, EdD, RD, LDN
Director, Didactic Program in
    Dietetics
Professor
Middle Tennessee University
Murfreesboro, TN

Margaret Tate, RDN, MS
Adjunct Faculty
Paradise Valley Community College
Phoenix, AZ

Jennifer L. Warren, MS, RD, LD
Instructor
The University of Akron
Akron, OH

PART I

The Past

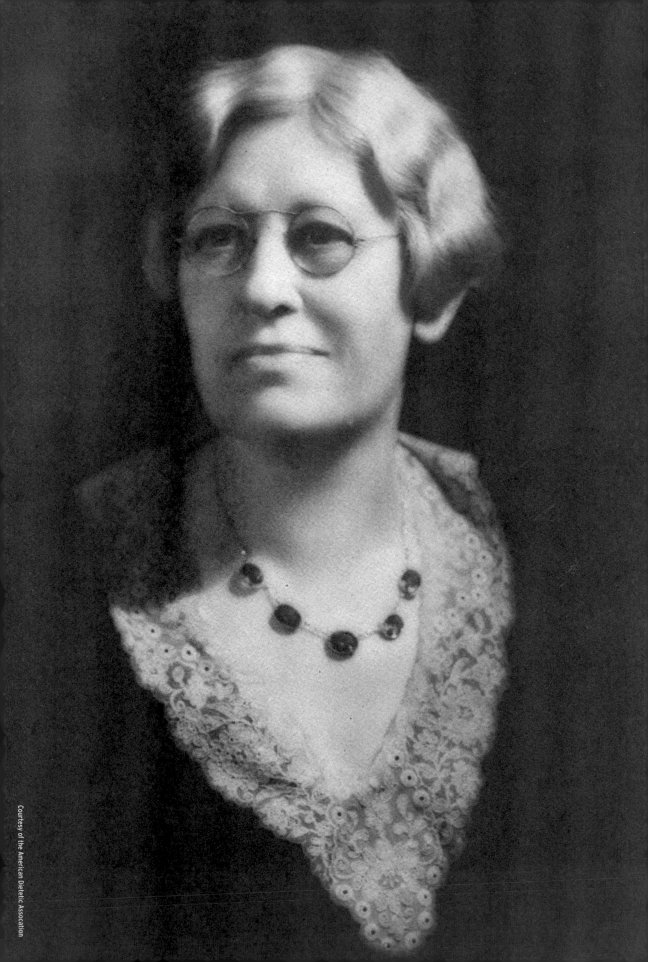

The Profession Is Born

The Very Beginning

When the professional association that represents most of the individuals practicing dietetics turns 100 in 2017, many will consider that it is also the 100th birthday of dietetics itself. These 100 years have been characterized by an ever-changing landscape. World events, legislation, social and economic changes, and scientific discoveries have all impacted the profession. With dynamic and dedicated leadership, the profession of dietetics has become a strong and viable career option.

So we begin with the history of the dietetics profession. History provides people with an opportunity to learn from past mistakes and can also show which of the seeds that were sown blossomed into successes and why. As stated on Radford University's Department of History website:

> The study of history is a window into the past that provides understanding of the present day, and how individuals, nations, and the global community might develop in the future. Historical study instructs how societies came to be and examines cultural, political, social, and economic influences across time and space.[1]

Prior to the establishment of the professional association 100 years ago, dietetic practice had an interesting, rich, and diverse past that stems from the much older history of food and health. Some very old sayings advise "An ounce of prevention is worth a pound of cure" and "An apple a day keeps the doctor away." The role of food in preventing, curing, treating, or causing illness has been recognized since the beginning of recorded human history. "If a man has pain inside, food and drink coming back to his mouth ... let him refrain from eating onions for three days" is the first known written dietary recommendation, carved on Babylonian stone tablets around 2500 B.C.[2] The typical daily regimen during this time consisted of barley paste or bread, onions, a few beans, and beer.

The Book of Judges in the Old Testament contains a prenatal dietary prescription that has withstood the test of time: "Therefore beware, and drink no wine or strong drink, and eat nothing unclean, for lo, you shall conceive and bear a son."[3] The Book of Daniel contains what is probably the first controlled dietary experiment. Daniel and the other young men from Judah asked their guards to allow them to maintain their ancestral traditions and eat pulses (legumes) and bread and drink water rather than the king's rich food and wine allowance for 10 days. At the end of the 10 days, they were healthier and better nourished than all the young men who had lived on the food assigned to them by the king.[4]

Scurvy, which is caused by a vitamin C deficiency, was described as early as 1500 B.C. in the Ebers Papyrus, and other descriptions appear in ancient Greek and Roman writings.[5] The word *diet* is from the Greek *diatta*, which means "manner of living."[6] It appears in many early writings, including those of Hippocrates and Galen.[7] The oldest known cookbook, Apicius's *De re Culinaria* (approximately 100 B.C.), contains many dietary principles that are still sound today.[8] One entire book of the 10 books contained in the cookbook attributed to Apicius is devoted to pulses, or legumes, which are mentioned in the Old Testament. In ancient China, food therapy was practiced as a special branch of medicine.[9] Chinese observations about diabetes date to the third century, and descriptions of night blindness and its correct dietary cure date to the seventh century.[10,11]

The Middle Ages

During the Song Dynasty (960–1279) in China, Ben Cao Tu Jing, in the *Atlas of Materia Medica* (1061), described a "clinical trial" to determine the efficacy of ginseng. He suggested, "In order to evaluate the efficacy of ginseng, find two people and let one eat ginseng and run, and the other run without ginseng. The one that did not eat ginseng will develop shortness of breath sooner."[12]

William the Conqueror was probably one of the first famous names in history to go on a weight-loss diet. In 1087, he tried to lose weight by going on a liquid diet, taking to his bed and consuming nothing but alcohol!

Hospital records from St. Bartholomew's Hospital (**Figure 1–1**), which was founded in Britain in 1123, provide the first written evidence of a typical hospital menu. Bread and beer formed the basis of the diet.[13] This obviously inadequate and unpalatable diet led to a prevalence of **scurvy** (a condition characterized by weakness, joint pain, skin lesions and bruising, bleeding gums, and loosening of teeth) among patients. Other conditions in early British hospitals were also poor. Sanitation was nonexistent, overcrowding was common, buildings were unsafe, and stern disciplinary measures were used on noncompliant patients.

With the publication of *De re Medicina* in 1478 in Florence, Italy, diet became an important part of medical practice. In this publication, medicine was divided into three branches: diseases treated manually, diseases treated by medicine, and diseases treated by diet. In 1480, the first printed cookbook appeared, containing reference to quality and varieties of meat, fish, fruits,

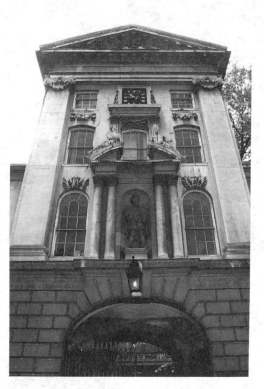

FIGURE 1–1 St. Bartholomew's Hospital, London.
Courtesy of Barts and the London NHS Trust

and vegetables; information on how they nourish the body; and directions on how they should be prepared.[14]

Weight-loss books appeared in the late 1600s to early 1700s. A Scotsman, Dr. George Cheyne, wrote two popular books, *An Essay of Health and Long Life* and *The English Malady*, in which he described a milk diet, which he claimed kept him "lank, fleet and nimble."[15]

Progress (?) in the Eighteenth and Nineteenth Centuries

The first hospitals in the United States were in Philadelphia—Philadelphia General Hospital was built in 1731, and Pennsylvania Hospital (**Figure 1–2**) was built in 1751.[13] In these hospitals, little thought was given to food, and conditions were very poor. Mush and molasses were the usual fare, with a pint of beer included for supper.[16] After the War of 1812, fruit was added to the menu as a garnish.

Until the eighteenth century, beliefs and writings about diet were based on insufficient scientific evidence. But with advances in chemistry and physics came the foundation necessary to establish dietetics as a profession. The work of Antoine-Laurent de Lavoisier (1743–1794) on digestion is generally regarded as the first modern, scientific research on nutrition (**Figure 1–3**). The son of a wealthy Parisian lawyer, Lavoisier was trained as a lawyer. Chemistry was his hobby.[17]

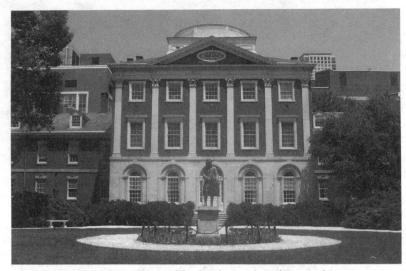

FIGURE 1–2 Pennsylvania Hospital, one of the first hospitals in the United States.
Copyright © 2006 by Sarah B. Hecht

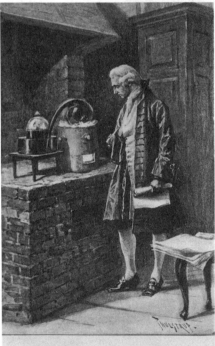

LAVOISIER IN HIS LABORATORY

FIGURE 1–3 Antoine Lavoisier is shown with the chemistry apparatus he used to study digestion.
Courtesy of the National Library of Medicine

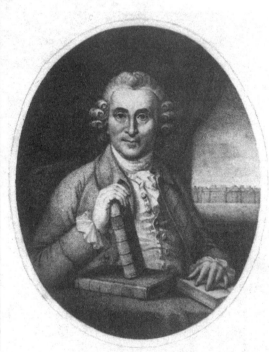

FIGURE 1–4 A portrait of James Lind holding his book Lind on Scurvy.
Courtesy of the Royal College of Physicians of Edinburgh

Nutritional epidemiology, the study of the relationship of diet to human disease, is often dated to 1747, the same year as the earliest known clinical trial was conducted by Dr. James Lind (**Figure 1–4**). Lind was the ship doctor on the HMS *Salisbury* when it set sail from England to the Plymouth Colony. During this time, scurvy and typhoid were often responsible for the deaths of more than half of the crewmembers of sailing ships. A British report in 1600 indicated that in the previous 20 years more than 10,000 mariners had died from scurvy alone. On board the *Salisbury*, Lind took 12 men ill with scurvy and divided them into six groups of two each. All ate the same food for breakfast, lunch, and dinner, but each group received a different supplement each day:

1. Quart of apple juice
2. Twenty-five drops of elixir vitriol (sulfuric acid and aromatics)
3. Two spoonfuls of vinegar three times a day
4. Concoction of herbs and spices
5. Half-pint of seawater daily
6. Two oranges and one lemon

The two men who ate the oranges and lemons recovered almost immediately. Both were fit enough to return to work in 6 days, and one became the nurse to the others. The two who drank the apple juice improved, but were not well enough to work. None of the others showed any improvement. Lind concluded that citrus fruit contained something that counteracted the ravages of scurvy; he gave all the men oranges and lemons, and they were cured. This discovery was followed by the development of a method for the concentration and preservation of citrus fruit juices for use at sea. In 1795, the British Royal Navy provided a daily ration of lemon or lime juice as an **antiscorbutic** (protects against scurvy). Because at the time both lemons and limes were called limes, Americans and Australians began to call English ships and sailors "lime-juicers," and later "limeys." Much later, a deficiency of vitamin C, ascorbic acid, was determined to be the cause of scurvy.[5]

Still, progress was slow. A patient in an English hospital in the eighteenth century would receive the only menu served each day:

- Four to five ounces of meat (usually already boiled for the broth)
- Three-quarters to one pound of bread
- Two to three pints of beer
- Pottage or pudding

Fruits and vegetables were missing from this daily allowance—they were suspected by some as being harmful and by others as having medicinal, rather than nutritive, value. Small amounts of cheese, butter, roots, and greens were sometimes included in the daily fare. Family and friends could bring food to supplement the meager hospital offerings, or patients could buy food from the food sellers who came through the wards.

The most expensive item on the menu was beer. Doctors at the time believed that alcohol was necessary to treat illness. Because water often was contaminated, beer was used extensively. When cost-cutting measures were instituted, the beer allowance was reduced or completely eliminated.

Patients who were unable to eat the full diet or who complained about the food were disciplined. Punishments included cutting the food allowance in half, omitting some meals entirely, or restricting patients to toast and water for a week.[18]

Meanwhile, famous individuals continued to go on diets, and other individuals became famous because of the diets they promoted. In 1811 the romantic poet Lord Byron reduced his weight from 194 to 130 pounds by drenching his food in vinegar. In the 1830s in the United States, the Reverend Sylvester Graham, nicknamed "Dr. Sawdust," railed against the sin of gluttony, which he said led to lust, indigestion, and the rearing of unhealthy children. His recommended Spartan diet included coarse, yeast-free, brown bread (including his famous Graham cracker), vegetables, and water.[15]

Little improvement in hospital conditions occurred until the humanitarian movement of the late nineteenth century. Great progress was made between 1850 and 1920.

Florence Nightingale (1820–1910) (**Figure 1–5**), a superintendent of nurses in British military hospitals in Turkey during the Crimean War (1854–1856), established foodservice for the troops. With the help of a French chef, Alexis Soyer, she reduced the death rate of injured soldiers by improving diet and sanitary conditions. Later, in her writings and nursing practice, Nightingale continued to demonstrate her belief in the importance of nutrition and foodservice management by emphasizing the selection and service of food and the art and science of feeding the sick.[19]

At around the same time, the low-carbohydrate, high-protein diet was first introduced. London undertaker William Banting lost 50 pounds on a high-protein regimen consisting of lean meat, dry toast, soft-boiled eggs, and vegetables. His 1864 book, *Letter on Corpulence*, became a bestseller, and by

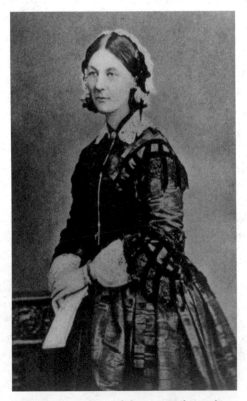

FIGURE 1–5 A portrait of Florence Nightingale.
Courtesy of Library of Congress, Prints & Photographs Division [reproduction number cph.3a09175]

1880 "Banting" had become the foremost American weight-loss strategy. Yet another proponent of high-protein diets, Dr. James Salisbury, recommended minced meat patties (what we know as Salisbury steaks) and hot water for improving health and aiding weight loss.[15]

The Iowa Agriculture School in Ames in 1872 was probably the first college to offer courses in cookery. A yearly course in "household chemistry," which included cookery, was started in 1877 at the Kansas State Agricultural College in Manhattan.[20] Other colleges and universities soon followed their lead.

In 1876 Dr. John Harvey Kellogg became the staff physician of the Battle Creek Sanitarium in Michigan. Kellogg invented granola and toasted flakes, for which his name is well known. At the time, he was known as a diet guru who crusaded for vegetarianism, pure foods, slow chewing, calorie counting, colon cleansing, and individualized diets.[15]

The first American dietitian is considered to be Sarah Tyson Rorer (1849–1937) (**Figure 1–6**). Her training consisted of some medical school lectures and a 3-month cooking course. In 1878 Rorer opened the Philadelphia Cooking School where students learned about food values, protein, and carbohydrates, but nothing about calories and vitamins. Students took 10 classes in chemistry, several in physiology and hygiene, and 10 on cooking for the sick. Twelve students graduated each year for 33 years, and they secured positions planning meals and supervising production in hospital kitchens.[21]

In 1877, the American Medical Association formed a Committee on Dietetics and asked Rorer to edit a new publication entitled *The Dietetic Gazette*.[22] Later, she published *Household News* on her own, in which she wrote articles on topics such as feeding the sick and designing a kitchen and answered readers' diet-related questions.[23] In her lifetime, she authored more than 50 books and booklets and wrote articles for such magazines as *Ladies' Home Journal*, *Table Talk*, and *Good Housekeeping*.[24] Rorer also established

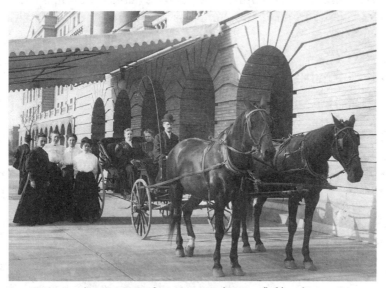

FIGURE 1–6 Sarah Tyson Rorer, first American dietitian (left) and Lenna Frances Cooper (right) in a carriage at the Battle Creek Sanitarium.
Courtesy of the Academy of Nutrition and Dietetics

the first diet kitchen and dietary counseling service, at the request of three well-known physicians.

Meanwhile the popular diets continued to evolve. Milk diets, earlier prescribed for indigestion and weight gain, now became popular for weight loss. Dr. Edward Hooker Dewey recommended skipping breakfast and a moderate fast as a weight-loss strategy. Other doctors of the time touted substituting carbohydrates with protein and limiting consumption of alcohol.[15]

Previously thought to be an infectious disease, beriberi received attention from several researchers around the world. In 1884, Kanehiro Takaki linked Japanese sailors' diet of polished rice to the disease **beriberi** (a condition characterized by weakness in the legs, hands, and arms and, later, weakening of the cardiac muscles, leading to heart failure). By adding milk and vegetables to the sailors' diet, he eliminated the disease.[25] In 1889, Christiaan Eijkman in the Dutch East Indies took the research one step further by proposing a nutritional hypothesis for the cause of beriberi. His experimentation with chickens led to the conclusion that unpolished rice contained an "anti-beriberi factor."[26] As with vitamin C, the identification of vitamin B_1 as the deficient nutrient came much later.

In 1896, the U.S. Department of Agriculture (USDA) published *Bulletin 28*, which featured the first food composition tables.[27] The *Bulletin* was an indispensable resource for dietetic practitioners for many years.

In 1898, when businessman Horace Fletcher was denied life insurance because of his weight, he lost 40 pounds by chewing every mouthful of food to liquefy it before swallowing. The slow-chewing movement (Fletcherism) took off, supported by diet guru Kellogg, whose patients were instructed to chew every mouthful of food 32 times before swallowing. This became known as "Fletcherizing."[15]

At the Lake Placid Conference on Home Economics in 1899, the term *dietitian* was first defined. The conference attendees determined that the title **dietitian** should be "applied to persons who specialize in the knowledge of food and can meet the demands of the medical profession for diet therapy."[28]

The Young Profession in the Twentieth Century

Florence Corbett established the first internship for dietitians in 1903 at the New York Department of Charities. Applicants for the 3-month course had to be older than 25 years of age, have 1 year of teaching experience, and be a domestic science graduate.[7]

In 1907, an English doctor, William Fletcher, conducted an experiment on inmates of a lunatic asylum in Kuala Lumpur, Malaysia, which provided definitive proof that certain types of rice were either the direct or indirect cause of beriberi. His experiment was rigorous and mimicked several features of a modern randomized trial.[26]

Working at the famed Lister Institute in London in 1912, Casimir Funk (1884–1967), a Polish-born biochemist, took Fletcher's thinking to the next level. He isolated the active substances in the husks of unpolished rice that were preventing beriberi and named them *amines*, because he believed they were derived from ammonia. Because these substances appeared essential for life, he added the prefix *vita*. Later, he postulated the existence of four such substances (B_1, B_2, C, and D), which he stated were necessary for normal health and for the prevention of deficiency diseases. Discovery and synthesis of all of the individual vitamins would come much later, but this initial discovery was a milestone in nutritional history.[29]

In 1910, dietitians were practicing in poorly defined roles with a diversity of titles. Few people could define the role of the *dietist, dietician, dietitian,* or *nutrition worker,* as dietitians were variously called. The title *nutritionist* appeared in the early 1920s, and the spelling of *dietitian* was agreed upon in 1930.[30]

Fighting faddism and quackery was an issue in 1910, just as it is today. Fletcherizing was just one example of a harmless but ineffective popular notion of that day. Calorie counting, high-protein or low-protein diets, and natural foods were other popular fads. Food scales, developed for diabetics, became central to diet plans.

Nutritional research received an unexpected boost in importance with the outbreak of World War I. The examination of 2.5 million military draftees in Great Britain in 1917 found 41% to be in poor health and unfit for duty, most commonly because of nutritional status.[31] In the United States, the American Red Cross enrolled dietitians for military duty. The initial qualifications were 2 years of college study majoring in home economics and 4 months of practical experience in hospital dietetics. The National Committee on Dietitian Service of the American Red Cross established these qualifications. The first military dietitian to serve overseas was deployed in May 1917. In World War I, 356 dietitians served in the armed services.[32] Mary Pascoe Huddleson, a dietitian with Base Hospitals No. 8, No. 117, and No. 214, was among them. Marjorie Hulsizer Copher was another dietitian who served overseas with Harvard U.S. Army Base Hospital No. 5, with British Expeditionary Force, May 1917–December 1918, and then with Base Hospital No. 57, American Expeditionary Force. She was decorated by King George V of England and by the French government for improving food services delivery systems in field hospitals and for introducing the relatively new profession of dietetics into the British Army. She later served as Chief Dietitian at Barnes Hospital in St. Louis. The highest honor bestowed by the Academy of Nutrition and Dietetics is named in her honor and described in Chapter 8.[33]

The nutritional expertise of these brave dietitians provided leadership for both the nourishment of hospitalized soldiers and the general public at home. Conservation of food was encouraged, and dietitians advised the government on efficient methods of food production, distribution, and preparation.

When the American Home Economic Association decided not to hold its annual meeting in 1917 because of the war, two dietitians, Lenna Frances Cooper (previously shown in **Figure 1–6**) and Lulu G. Graves (**Figure 1–7**), organized a special meeting of hospital dietitians to discuss emergency war needs. Out of the meeting of 98 people, the American Dietetic Association (ADA) was formed (**Figure 1–8**). This association, with 39 charter members and dues of $1 per year, was formed to address the interests of dietitians. Its

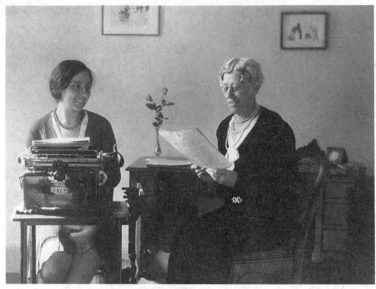

FIGURE 1–7 Lulu Graves, first president of the ADA, now known as the Academy of Nutrition and Dietetics, in her office with her assistant.
Courtesy of the Academy of Nutrition and Dietetics

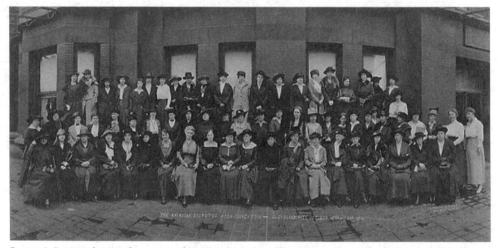

FIGURE 1–8 Attendees at the 1917 conference where the ADA, now known as the Academy of Nutrition and Dietetics, was founded.
Courtesy of the Academy of Nutrition and Dietetics

first president was Lulu Graves, who was head of the department at Lakeside Hospital in Cleveland (**Figure 1–9**). The first meeting of the ADA (now known as the Academy of Nutrition and Dietetics) was held in the basement at Lakeside Hospital. Graves served as president for the first 3 years. Lenna Frances Cooper served as the first vice president.[7]

In 1918, *Diet and Health with a Key to the Calories*, written by the best-known and best-loved woman physician in America—Dr. Lulu Hunt Peters—was a bestseller. The diet began with a fast and then transitioned to Fletcherism and calorie counting, with a 1,200-calorie-a-day regimen prescribed for life.[15]

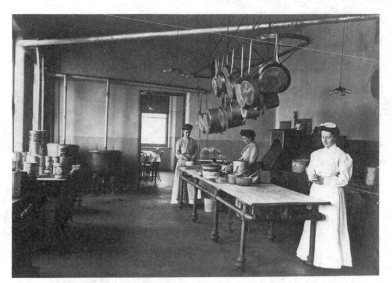

FIGURE 1–9 Lakeside Hospital kitchen, 1905. The first meeting of the American Dietetic Association was held in the basement of this hospital in 1917.
Courtesy of the Academy of Nutrition and Dietetics

Dieto-therapy as practiced in the early 1900s consisted of many special diets, such as the Sippy Diet for ulcers, which consisted of cream and poached eggs. Diabetic diets varied widely, even after the discovery of insulin in 1921. Doctors prescribed very-low-calorie diets of 600 to 750 calories a day for severely obese patients beginning in 1928. Ten years later, the regimen was reduced to 400 calories a day.

The 1920s saw a dizzying array of food-limiting regimens. The 18-day Hollywood diet allowed 585 calories a day, limited mostly to grapefruit, oranges, eggs, and Melba toast. The lamb chop and the pineapple diets were also popular. The first food-combining diet was introduced, in which dieters were admonished not to combine starches, fruits, and proteins in the same meal.[15]

On a more scientific level, the successful treatment of pernicious anemia with a special diet was reported in the *Journal of the American Medical Association*.[34] The passage of the federal Maternity and Infancy Act in the 1920s allowed state health departments to employ nutritionists.[30] The passage of Title V of the Social Security Act in 1935 provided major impetus for the employment of nutrition consultants in state and local health departments by making federal funds available for this purpose.[30,35]

In 1922, the Medical Department Professional Service School at Walter Reed General Hospital was established, becoming the first Army training program for dietitians. The program met ADA requirements and was the only training course provided for dietitians by the Army from 1922 to 1942 (**Figure 1–10**). World War II contributed to the public recognition of the role of dietitians. Nearly 2,000 dietitians were commissioned in the armed services, and many others educated the public at home. The practice of dietetics broadened to include institutions such as restaurants, airlines, and industrial plants. After the war, dietitians were granted full military status, and their

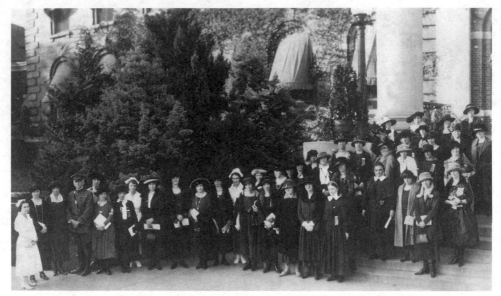

FIGURE 1–10 Dietitians at Walter Reed General Hospital in 1922.
Courtesy of the Academy of Nutrition and Dietetics

position in the healthcare setting was strengthened with the emphasis on allied health professions and the healthcare team concept.[7]

Passage of the National School Lunch Act in 1946 expanded dietetics to include the establishment of school lunch programs, including the training of personnel in foodservice and nutrition education. The Hill-Burton Hospital Facilities Survey and Construction Act (1946) and the Medicare and Medicaid legislation of the 1960s created demand for the services of consultant dietitians in healthcare facilities such as nursing homes.[35]

In 1948, Take Off Pounds Sensibly (TOPS) became the first national group dieting organization. The TOPS program focused on calories, scales, food diaries, and mutual support. Still going strong, TOPS has added physical activity and the use of exchange lists to its weight-loss program.[15]

Dietitians were actively recruited for service during the Korean War (**Figure 1–11**). At this time, the role of the military dietitian started to expand to include not only therapeutic dietetics, but also the supervision and operation of the entire hospital foodservice.[32]

Overeaters Anonymous was founded in 1960 and Weight Watchers in 1961. During this same time, Mead Johnson introduced a diet formula, Metrecal, whose success spawned many imitators. The 1960s saw a number of diet book bestsellers. Touting the low-carbohydrate, high-protein diets were *Calories Don't Count* and *The Doctor's Quick Weight Loss Diet*. In the alcohol-friendly, low-carbohydrate category were *The Drinking Man's Diet* and *Martinis and Whipped Cream*.[15]

The civil rights movement of the 1960s brought the issues of poverty and hunger into the political spotlight. The government instituted its war on poverty, and Senator Hubert Humphrey worked with the Senate Select Committee on Nutrition and Human Needs.[36] As a result of these and other efforts, USDA food assistance programs to low-income families were established or

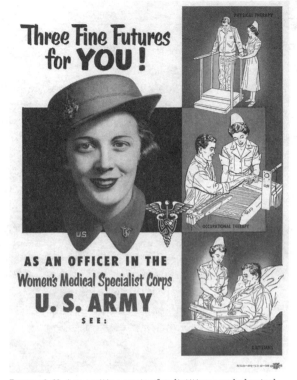

FIGURE 1–11 A recruiting poster for dietitians and physical and occupational therapists during the Korean War.
Women's Medical Specialist Corps recruiting poster. U.S. War Poster Collection (MSSO44), Betty H. Carter Women Veterans Historical Project, University of North Carolina at Greensboro, NC, USA

expanded in the 1970s. Important among these were the Food Stamp Program and school lunch and breakfast programs; child care and summer food-service for children; supplemental feeding programs for Women, Infants, and Children (WIC); and nutrition for the elderly.[37]

During the Vietnam conflict, 26 Army dietitians were assigned to all four combat tactical zones. They formulated meals for hospital patients on modified diets, planned the basic troop-issue menus for all Army personnel in the country, and implemented the menus for all personnel in medical treatment facilities. These tasks were complicated by the fact that in 1966 there were 385,000 troops in Vietnam and refrigeration was minimal. Air Force dietitians developed a system to order, prepare, and serve therapeutic in-flight meals for patients who were being evacuated from combat zones.[38]

Food assistance programs have developed more rapidly and with more support than nutrition education programs. In 1968, the Cooperative Extension Service of the USDA began the Expanded Food and Nutrition Education Program (EFNEP), which provides nutrition and food education for low-income families. In 1975, 3 years after the start of the WIC program, an education component was legislated. And, in 1977, nutrition education was incorporated into the Food Stamp Program. The Food and Agriculture Act of 1977 included the Nutrition Education and Training Program (NETP or NET), the first federal nutrition program for children.[36]

TABLE 1–1	
Timeline of Late-Twentieth-Century Diets	
1970s	Astronauts' diet—liquid meals.
1972	Dr. Atkins' Diet Revolution—lots of meat. Carbohydrates are banned.
1976	The Last Chance Diet—fasting and liquid drinks made from animal tendons and hides. Fifty-eight deaths were attributed to these and similar liquid formulas that lack essential nutrients.
1978	Scarsdale Diet—high protein, 700 calories per day.
1979	Pritikin Program for Diet and Exercise—very-low-fat regimen.
1981	The Beverly Hills Diet—food-combining diet with lots of fruit.
1983	Jenny Craig is founded.
1992	Dr. Atkins' New Diet Revolution.
1993	Eat More, Weigh Less—low-fat, vegetarian diet.
1995	The Zone—low-carbohydrate, high-protein diet soon joined by Sugar Busters, Protein Power, and The Carbohydrate Addicts' Diet.
1996	The New Beverly Hills Diet (see 1981).
1998	Lose Weight with Apple Vinegar—Lord Byron's strategy resurfaces!
1999	Dr. Atkins publishes yet another revision.

The Academy of Nutrition and Dietetics and others expressed the need for making nutrition education a primary component of all food assistance programs.[39]

As the general public continued to seek ways to lose weight quickly and easily, a steady stream of diet books rolled off the presses (**Table 1–1**). Most were slight variations on old themes.

Entering the Twenty-First Century

In 2003, *The South Beach Diet* hit the bookstores. It is a moderate diet falling midway between the low-fat, high-carbohydrate recommendations of trained dietitians and the low-carbohydrate, high-protein Atkins diet.

Today, dietetics is an honored profession with members striving to achieve the highest professional standards of integrity, service, competence, and vision. Two leaders of the profession wrote recently:

> *Our profession today is marked by achievement and change.... [We] have come a long way in a relatively short period of time. We have become valued professional members of health-care teams and recognized experts in food and nutrition, foodservice management, and wellness.... We need the courage to perceive ourselves succeeding in new roles, to attract a diversity of people to dietetics, and to polish and practice marketing, management, leadership, and sales skills.*[40]

Change is occurring rapidly in all areas of the dietetics profession—education, research, and practice. At an address to the ADA in 2003, the Surgeon General of the United States, Richard Carmona, commended the professional association for its leadership in advancing healthcare quality through nutrition. One of his main priorities as surgeon general was disease prevention. He stated that 7 out of 10 Americans who die each year die of a chronic disease, most of which are preventable by relatively simple steps: healthy eating, being active, and not smoking. Current efforts to encourage Americans to adopt healthy behaviors to prevent disease have not been successful. One of the reasons for this failure is low health literacy. **Health literacy** is an individual's ability to access, understand, and use health-related information and services to make appropriate health decisions. The inadequacy of nutrition education in medical schools is another concern, as 8 of the 10 leading diseases in the United States are linked to nutrition.[41]

The surgeon general challenged dietitians to make sure that their patients understand what they can do to stay healthy. He said:

> *Nutrition education is your business! Every single day you translate complex nutrition principles into an array of healthy eating options for the American public ... your expertise is valued at the highest levels. Wherever you are—in clinics, hospitals, outpatient or long-term care settings, in sports, education or the restaurant and food industry—your work is tremendously important to the health and well-being of Americans. And your work is becoming more and more important as we move towards a national prevention agenda. We need you—your passion, your expertise and your experience as nutrition professionals.*[41]

A recent president of the Academy of Nutrition and Dietetics stated that trends toward preventive care and people's interest in achieving and maintaining an overall healthy lifestyle are two of the most dramatic developments affecting dietetics in the last two decades. To best adapt to these positive changes, she advised dietitians to sharpen their professional skills, gain deeper understanding of the unique needs of diverse populations, use critical-thinking skills to solve the difficult problems facing their communities, and seek opportunities for leadership.[42]

The priority areas at this time are aging, child nutrition, healthcare reform, nutrigenomics, sustainability, medical nutritional therapy, nutritional monitoring, nutrition research, obesity, and state government issues related to dietetics. Other food and nutrition areas of current importance are hunger, food insecurity, HIV/AIDS, food safety, allied health, and physical activity.

On January 1, 2012, the ADA officially became the Academy of Nutrition and Dietetics. The name change was enacted to better reflect the strong science background and academic expertise of members and the academy's mission, vision, philosophy, and values.[43] The following year, in 2013, the optional credential registered dietitian nutritionist (RDN) was approved for registered dietitians (RDs).[44] And in 2014, dietetic technicians, registered (DTRs) were allowed to begin using nutrition and dietetics technician registered (NDTR).[45] Both were approved to better reflect to consumers who these professionals are and what they do.

Summary

Although there is a long history of the relationship of food to health, the profession of dietetics is very young. Much of the progress in the profession has been made in the last 100 years (**Table 1–2**). Advances in scientific research, legislation, social and economic factors, military conflicts, and the leadership of some dynamic and dedicated dietitians have contributed to the advancement of the profession.

"Remember the 'old girls,' as they made it possible for us to work for our dream." This statement was made by Marion Mason, PhD, RD, Ruby Winslow Professor of Nutrition, Emerita, at Simmons College in Boston, in an address to the Massachusetts Dietetic Association.[46] It was Lulu Graves, the first president of the ADA, who first sounded the call for teamwork between physicians and dietitians. "The future of dietetics is assured. It is the privilege of those of us who are now in the work to conduct it along such lines that, in the not very distant future, it will be recognized as part of the medical team."[47] That time has arrived!

TABLE 1–2

A Timeline of Selected Milestones in Dietetic History

2500 B.C.	Avoidance of onions is the first known dietary prescription.
1500 B.C.	Nutrient deficiency disease, scurvy, is described.
100 B.C.	Apicius's *De re Culinaria* is the first known cookbook.
1061	Ben Cao Tu Jing tests efficacy of ginseng.
1087	William the Conqueror goes on liquid diet to lose weight.
1123	St. Bartholomew's Hospital, London, is founded.
1478	*De re Medicina* is published in Florence, Italy. Diet becomes part of medical practice.
1480	First cookbook is printed.
1731	First hospital in United States is built in Philadelphia, Pennsylvania.
1747	James Lind conducts clinical trial on scurvy patients.
1792	Lavoisier outlines process of the "physiology of nutrition."
1811	Lord Byron uses vinegar to lose weight.
1854	Florence Nightingale uses nutrition to reduce death rate of soldiers.
1864	William Banting's bestseller touts high-protein diet for weight loss.
1872	Iowa Agricultural School offers courses in cookery.
1876	Dr. John Harvey Kellogg develops toasted flakes and granola.
1877	Kansas State offers course in household chemistry, and the American Medical Association forms committee on dietetics.
1878	Sarah Tyson Rorer opens Philadelphia Cooking School.
1884	Kanehiro Takaki adds milk and vegetables to Japanese sailors' diet of polished rice in order to cure beriberi.
1889	Christiaan Eijkman proposes nutritional hypothesis for beriberi.
1896	USDA publishes first food composition tables.
1898	Horace Fletcher proposes "Fletcherizing" for weight loss.
1899	The title of *dietitian* is defined.

1903	New York Department of Charities offers the first dietetic internship.
1907	William Fletcher conducts randomized trial on cause of beriberi.
1912	Casimir Funk isolates "vitamins" and suggests that dietary deficiencies of vitamins cause beriberi, rickets, pellagra, sprue, and other diseases.
1914	World War I boosts impetus for nutrition research.
1917	The American Dietetic Association is founded.
1920	Title nutritionist first appears, and the Maternity and Infancy Act allows states to employ nutritionists.
1921	Insulin is discovered.
1930	Spelling of *dietitian* is agreed upon.
1933	Robert R. Williams synthesizes and names vitamin B_1.
1935	Title V of the Social Security Act—federal funding for nutrition positions.
1938	Conrad Elvehjem identifies niacin as the missing nutrient causing pellagra.
1939	World War II contributes to public recognition of dietitians.
1946	National School Lunch Act expands dietetics to include school lunches.
1947	First national dieting group is founded—TOPS.
1960	Overeaters Anonymous is founded.
1961	Weight Watchers is founded.
1968	Expanded food and nutrition education programs for low-income families.
1969	Registration of dietitians is begun.
1972	Women, Infants, and Children (WIC) program is started.
1975	Nutrition education program added to WIC.
1977	Food and Agriculture Act includes a nutrition education component.
1983	Certification of dietetic technicians is begun.
1993	Specialty board certification for RDs is started.
1999	Registration exams first administered by computer.
2010	2009 Code of Ethics for the Profession of Dietetics goes into effect.
2012	American Dietetic Association becomes the Academy of Nutrition and Dietetics.
2013	RDN title option for RDs approved.
2014	NDTR title option approved for DTRs.

The increasing diversity of the profession through the years has created the need to broaden the focus of this goal. The ADA was founded at a time when most dietitians worked in acute-care hospitals. Just 32% of dietitians and 44% of dietetic technicians are now employed in this setting.[48] At the beginning of the twenty-first century, Lulu Graves's quote could be modified to read: It is the privilege of those of us who are now in the work to conduct it along such lines that, in the not very distant future, it will be recognized as the best source for nutrition information and the professionals as those best trained to help consumers make individualized food choices. This comprehensive goal is exemplified in the words inscribed on the Academy of Nutrition and Dietetics seal, adopted in 1940, *Quam Plurimis Prodesse*—"to benefit as many as possible."

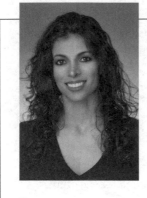

Profile of a Professional

Natalie Petro, RD, LD, CLC

Lead Dietitian
Women, Infants, and Children (WIC) Program. Located in Norcross, Georgia

Education
BS in Nutrition and Food Science, Georgia Southern University, Statesboro, Georgia
Dietetic Internship, Georgia Department of Public Health, Atlanta, Georgia

How did you first hear about dietetics and decide to become a registered dietitian nutritionist?
I have always loved food, people, and fitness, but I did not know about dietetics when starting college. I began college in a nursing program. Part of the nursing curriculum included a nutrition course. My nutrition professor was so enthusiastic about nutrition and how it impacted life! That class was one of the only classes I enjoyed in the nursing curriculum. I subsequently decided that nursing was not for me. Nutrition incorporated everything I loved. I transferred in-state to another school that had a dietetics major, and the rest is history!

What was your route to registration?
I started college at the University of Alabama in Tuscaloosa but transferred and graduated with a BS in Nutrition and Food Science from Georgia Southern University. I completed the Georgia Department of Public Health dietetic internship.

Are you involved in any professional organizations?
I am currently an Academy of Nutrition and Dietetics member and serve at the state level on the Nutrition Education Committee and Nutrition Task Force.

What has been your career path in dietetics, and what are you doing now?
I have worked for the Women, Infants, and Children (WIC) program for 8 years. Currently I serve WIC families as Lead Dietitian.

What excites you about dietetics and the future of our profession?
I am passionate about serving people. Dietetics is the one profession that gives you the opportunity to make an impact through prevention, meet people where they are, and encourage constant progress to maximize quality of life. The science of nutrition, tools, and techniques are constantly changing so RDNs are always learning. The more you learn, the more you want to learn! As you learn, you start to see how nutrition fits into the bigger picture of health and how it all connects. Working for something bigger than yourself is the most rewarding experience.

How is teamwork important to you in your position? How have you been involved in team projects?
I rely heavily on my colleagues. One person cannot know everything, so recognizing your colleagues' strengths and their areas of expertise helps you to know who to call on if you need help or advice so you can best serve your clients. Working with great colleagues increases your knowledge and experience in every area. We collaborate daily with healthcare professionals to develop a common plan of care for the families we serve to maximize the effectiveness of our interventions. Dietitians working closely with physicians, nurses, and other health professionals bring a variety of perspectives, techniques, and tools to treating a problem, not just the symptoms.

What words of wisdom do you have for future dietetics professionals?
Aim to be a part of something bigger than yourself. To serve and contribute to something like that is more amazing than you can imagine! Do not limit yourself. Continue

to learn and grow wherever you are. The more you learn and grow, the more opportunity God has to use you in His plan to make an impact, changing you and those you serve in the process. Never be too busy for people or too busy to listen. Life is too short, so serve wholeheartedly. Make your profession your passion. Lastly, "Be the kind of person when your feet hit the floor in the morning the Devil says, 'Oh no! They're up!'" (Dwayne Johnson).

Suggested Activities

1. Search the Internet to find additional contributions Lavoisier made to the practice of dietetics, specifically in the areas of food hygiene and hospital sanitation.

2. The James Lind Library has been created to introduce people to the characteristics of fair tests of medical treatments. Visit the Library's website (www.jameslindlibrary.org) to find out the characteristics of a "fair test." Compare your findings to the definition of the scientific method.

3. Use the Internet to research the history of pellagra. When was it determined that pellagra was a vitamin deficiency disease? Who made this discovery? Which vitamin was missing from the diets of those who became ill with pellagra? Why was this vitamin not present in their diet?

4. What are the most recent developments within the dietetics profession? Visit the website of the Academy of Nutrition and Dietetics (www .eatright.org) to read the latest news. Read the press releases and list five of the most significant recent developments within the profession.

5. How does dietetic practice differ in other countries? Do an Internet search to compare international dietetic associations.

6. Many of the weight-loss regimens listed in this chapter would be considered "quackery." Visit www.quackwatch.com to see what is being done today to combat such practices.

7. Read one of the autobiographies in *Legends and Legacies* (C. E. Vickery and N. Cotugna, Kendall/Hunt Publishing, 1990) and give an oral report to your class.

8. Secure a very old book on health or cooking from a library or used bookstore. Compare its content to present-day beliefs and practices.

9. Interview a 50-year member of the profession to obtain a personal history of changes that have occurred in the dietetics profession.

10. Read a journal article chronicling the history of dietetic practice during World War I or II. Two examples are:
    - Hodges PA. Perspective on history: military dietetics in Europe during World War I. *J Am Diet Assoc.* 1993;93:897–900.
    - Hodges PA. Perspective on history: military dietetics in the Philippines during World War II. *J Am Diet Assoc.* 1992;92:840–843.

Selected Websites

- www.chemheritage.org—The Chemical Heritage Foundation fosters an understanding of chemistry's impact on society.
- www.eatright.org—The Academy of Nutrition and Dietetics is the world's largest organization of food and nutrition professionals.
- www.jameslindlibrary.org—The James Lind Library seeks to help people understand the fair tests of treatments in healthcare.
- www.prbm.com—The Philadelphia Rare Books and Manuscripts Company offers a variety of old and rare nutrition- and health-related books.

Suggested Readings

Banting FG, Best CH, Collip JB, Campbell WR, Fletcher AA. Pancreatic extracts in the treatment of diabetes mellitus. *Can Med Assoc J.* 1922;12:141–146.

Fletcher W. Rice and beri-beri: preliminary report on an experiment conducted in the Kuala Lumpur Insane Asylum. *Lancet.* 1907;1:1776–1779.

Fraser L. *Losing It: America's Obsession with Weight and the Industry That Feeds on It.* New York: EP Dutton; 1997.

Funk C. *The Vitamines.* Authorized translation from 2nd German ed. by Dubin HE. Baltimore: Williams & Wilkins; 1922.

Mestel R. Round and round we go. *Los Angeles Times,* December 29, 2003, Section F, p. 1.

Stearns P. *Fat History.* New York: New York University Press; 2002.

Vickery C, Cotugna N. *Legends and Legacies.* Dubuque, IA: Kendall/Hunt Publishing; 1990.

References

1. Why study history? Radford University Department of History website. Available at: http://www.radford.edu/content/chbs/home/history/why-history.html. Accessed January 21, 2016.
2. Jastrow M. *The Civilization of Babylonia and Assyria.* Philadelphia: JB Lippincott; 1915.
3. *The Bible* (Revised Standard Version), Judges 13:14. New York: Collins; 1971.
4. *The Bible* (Revised Standard Version), Daniel 1:5–16. New York: Collins; 1971.
5. Huskey RJ. A simple experiment on scurvy. Available at: http://www.ca-biomed.org/csbr/pdf/nut.pdf. Accessed January 21, 2016.
6. Gove PB, ed. *Webster's Third New International Dictionary.* Springfield, MA: G & C Merriam; 1971.
7. Barber MI, ed. *History of the American Dietetic Association (1917–1959).* Philadelphia: JB Lippincott; 1959.
8. Vehling JD, trans. *Apicius: Cooking and Dining in Imperial Rome.* Chicago: Walter M. Hill; 1936.
9. Whang J. Chinese traditional food therapy. *J Am Diet Assoc.* 1981;78:55–57.

10. Durant W. *Our Oriental Heritage*. New York: Simon & Schuster; 1935.

11. Garrison FH. *An Introduction to the History of Medicine*, 4th ed. Philadelphia: WB Saunders; 1967.

12. Cao Tu Jing B. *Atlas of Materia Medica*. Collected and edited by Shang Z. Anhui, China: Anhui Science and Technology Press (in Chinese); 1994.

13. Isch C. A history of hospital fare. In: Beeuwkes AM, Todhunter EN, Weigley ES, eds. *Essays on the History of Nutrition and Dietetics*. Chicago: The American Dietetic Association; 1967.

14. De Honesta Voluptate. In: Whitcomb M, ed. *Literary Source Book of the Italian Renaissance*. Philadelphia; 1900.

15. Swartz H. *Never Satisfied*. New York: Free Press; 1986.

16. The American Dietetic Association Study Commission on Dietetics. *A New Look at the Profession of Dietetics*. Chicago: The American Dietetic Association; 1984.

17. Needham J. Clerks and craftsmen in China and the West. In: *Lectures and Addresses on the History of Science and Technology*. Cambridge, MA: Cambridge University Press; 1970.

18. Rabenn WB. Hospital diets in eighteenth century England. In: Beeuwkes AM, Todhunter EN, Weigley ES, eds. *Essays on the History of Nutrition and Dietetics*. Chicago: The American Dietetic Association; 1967.

19. Cooper LF. Florence Nightingale's contribution to dietetics. In: Beeuwkes AM, Todhunter EN, Weigley ES, eds. *Essays on the History of Nutrition and Dietetics*. Chicago: The American Dietetic Association; 1967.

20. Gilson HE. Some historical notes on the development of diet therapy. In: Beeuwkes AM, Todhunter EN, Weigley ES, eds. *Essays on the History of Nutrition and Dietetics*. Chicago: The American Dietetic Association; 1967.

21. Cooper LF. The dietitian and her profession. *J Am Diet Assoc*. 1938;4:751–758.

22. Rorer ST. Early dietetics. *J Am Diet Assoc*. 1934;x:289.

23. Rorer ST. Feeding the sick. *Household News*. 1893;1:69; Rorer ST. How to design a kitchen. *Household News*. 1894;2:17; Rorer ST. Answers to inquiries. *Household News*. 1893;1:13.

24. Weigley ES. Sarah Tyson Rorer. First American dietitian? *J Am Diet Assoc*. 1980;77:11–15.

25. Jikei University School of Medicine. Founding Spirit—Patient-Centered Medical Care. Available at: http://www.jikei.ac.jp/eng/found.html. Accessed March 17, 2016.

26. Vandenbroucke JP. The contribution of William Fletcher's 1907 report to finding a cause and cure for beriberi. The James Lind Library. Available at: http://www.jameslindlibrary.org/articles/the-contribution-of-william-fletchers-1907-report-to-finding-a-cause-and-cure-for-beriberi/. Accessed January 21, 2016.

27. Atwater WO, Bryant AF. *The Chemical Composition of American Food Materials*. U.S. Department of Agriculture Bulletin No. 28. Washington, DC: U.S. Government Printing Office; 1896.

28. Corbett FR. The training of dietitians for hospitals. *J Home Econ*. 1909;1:62.

29. Funk C. The etiology of the deficiency diseases. *J State Med*. 1912;341–368.

30. Egan M. Public health nutrition services: issues today and tomorrow. *J Am Diet Assoc*. 1980;77:423.

31. Burnett J. *Plenty and Want: A Social History of Diet in England from 1815 to the Present Day*. London: Nelson; 1966.

32. Baylor University. History of Military Dietitians. Available at: http://www.baylor.edu/graduate/nutrition/index.php?id=68073. Accessed January 21, 2016.

33. The Academy of Nutrition and Dietetics. The Marjorie Hulsizer Copher Award. Available at: http://www.eatright.org. Accessed September 30, 2015.

34. Minot GR, Murphy WP. Treatment of pernicious anaemia by a special diet. *JAMA*. 1926;87:470–476.

35. Eliot MM, Heseltine MM. Nutrition in maternal and child health programs. *Nutr Rev*. 1947:533–535.

36. Bray GA. Nutrition in the Humphrey tradition. *J Am Diet Assoc*. 1979;75:116–121.

37. Cross AT. USDA's strategies for the 80s: nutrition education. *J Am Diet Assoc.* 1980;76:333–337.

38. Ritchie Hartwick, AM. Army Medical Specialist Corps in Vietnam. Available at: www .vietnamwomensmemorial.org/pdf/ahartwick.pdf. Accessed January 21, 2016.

39. ADA testifies in favor of improving USDA domestic feeding programs. *ADA Courier.* 1993;32:2.

40. Calvert-Finn S, Rinke W. Probing the envelope of dietetics by transforming challenges into opportunities. *J Am Diet Assoc.* 1980;89:1441–1443.

41. Carmona RH. Remarks at ADA's 2003 Food & Nutrition Conference and Expo, San Antonio, TX, October 27, 2003.

42. Smith Edge M. Remarks at ADA's 2003 Food & Nutrition Conference & Expo, San Antonio, TX, October 27, 2003.

43. Academy of Nutrition and Dietetics. Press Release: American Dietetic Association Officially Becomes the Academy of Nutrition and Dietetics. Available at: http://www.eatright .org. Accessed January 3, 2012.

44. The Academy of Nutrition and Dietetics. RDN Credential: Frequently Asked Questions. Available at: http://www.eatright.org. Accessed September 30, 2015.

45. The Academy of Nutrition and Dietetics. NDTR Credential: Frequently Asked Questions—DPD Program Graduates, August 2014. Available at: http://www.eatright .org. Accessed September 30, 2015.

46. Fitz PA. President's page: About 80 years ago…. *J Am Diet Assoc.* 1997;97:1160–1161.

47. Cassell JA. *Carry the Flame: The History of the American Dietetic Association.* Chicago: The American Dietetic Association; 1990.

48. Academy of Nutrition and Dietetics. *2013 Compensation and Benefits Survey of the American Dietetic Association.* Chicago: Academy of Nutrition and Dietetics; 2014.

The Present

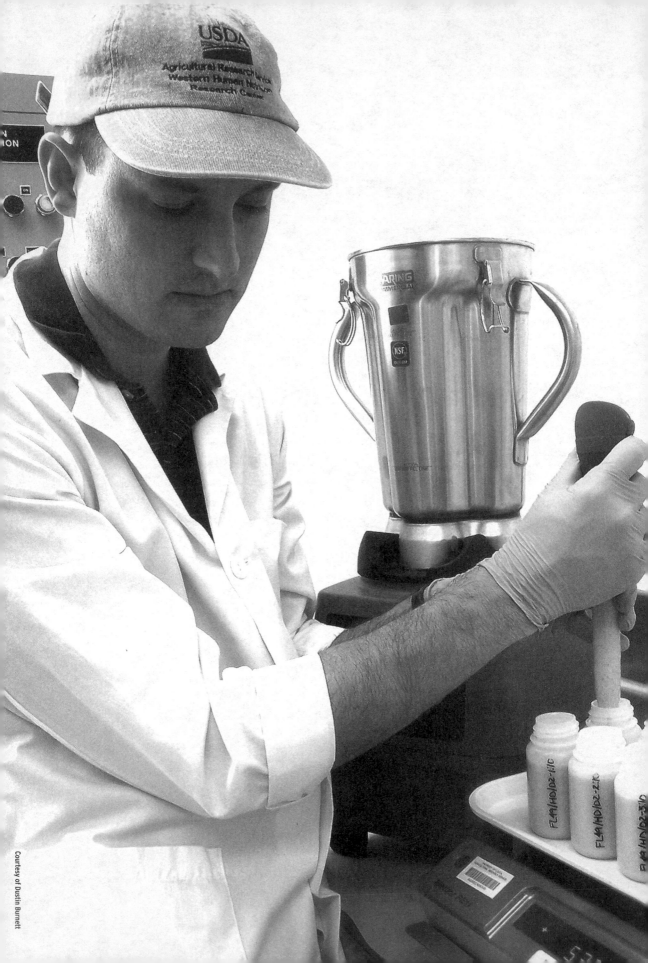

The Dietetics Profession

"To benefit as many as possible" appeared on the seal of the American Dietetic Association (and is still in use today on the seal of the Academy of Nutrition and Dietetics). It is an even more relevant goal of the profession today than it was in 1940 when it was first adopted. The scope of professional practice is continuously widening, and the knowledge base of nutrition is deepening. Since that first meeting in Cleveland in 1917, the Academy of Nutrition and Dietetics has grown to be the largest food and nutrition organization in the world. This growth has occurred because of members who are willing to seize and/or create opportunities and who have solid educational foundations that are diverse enough to allow practice in a myriad of areas.

What is dietetics? What makes it a profession? Who are today's dietitians? Where do they work, and what do they do? What kind of compensation and benefits do they enjoy in their positions, and what are some of the issues facing the profession today? These are the questions that are addressed in this chapter (**Figure 2–1**).

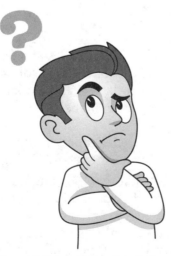

FIGURE 2–1 Just what is dietetics?

What Is Dietetics?

At the center of the professional association seal, adopted in 1940, are images representing the three main characteristics of the profession: a balance, representing science as the foundation of dietetics; a caduceus, representing the close relationship between dietetics and medicine; and a cooking vessel, representing cooking and food preparation. Surrounding this is a shaft of wheat, representing bread as the staff of life; acanthus leaves, representing growth and life; and a cornucopia, representing an abundant food supply. The name of the association and its founding date in Roman numerals are printed around the edge. The seal appears on registration certificates for registered dietitians and for registered dietetic technicians and on the gold member pin. Consider the following definitions of *dietetics*:

- "The scientific study of food preparation and intake."[1]
- "The science of applying nutritional principles to the planning and preparation of foods and regulation of the diet in relation to both health and disease."[2]

These definitions are woefully inadequate for what dietetics has grown to become. The basis of dietetics is the firm belief that optimal nutrition is essential for the health and well-being of every person. This is why dietetics is an integral component of the healthcare field. A team effort by doctors, nurses, and dietitians is usually necessary to return a patient to health. However, it is possible that no other profession offers such a diversity of opportunities outside of the traditional healthcare arena as the field of dietetics. Early dietetic practitioners were usually found in an institutional kitchen—for which the dictionary definitions would have been adequate. Today, dietitians can be found almost anywhere. For this reason, a recent survey of dietetics made use of a very broad definition of *dietetics*:

> A *dietetics-related position is considered to be any position that requires or makes use of your education, training, and/or experience in dietetics or nutrition, including situations outside of "traditional" dietetics practice.*[3]

What Is a Profession?

A general definition of a *profession* might be "an occupation for which preliminary training is intellectual in character, involving knowledge and learning as distinguished from mere skill, which is pursued largely for others and not merely for oneself and in which financial return is not an accepted measure of success."[4]

The Goals Committee of the Academy of Nutrition and Dietetics interprets a profession as a calling requiring the following:

- Specialized knowledge and often long and intensive preparation
- Maintenance, by force of organization or concerted opinion, of high standards of achievement and conduct
- Instruction in skills and methods as well as scientific, historical, or scholarly principles underlying such skills and methods

- Commitment of its members to continued study
- A kind of work that has as its primary purpose the rendering of a public service[5]

A professional is one who represents or belongs to a profession.

How Is Dietetics a Profession?

Five main characteristics of dietetic practice qualify it for professional status:

1. A specialized body of knowledge
2. Specialized services rendered to society
3. An obligation for service to the client that overrides personal considerations
4. Concern for competence and honor among the practitioners
5. An obligation to continuing education, research, and sharing of knowledge for the common good[6]

What Is a Registered Dietitian Nutritionist?

A dietitian has been defined as "a professional person who is a translator of the science and art of foods, nutrition, and dietetics in the service of people—whether individually or in families or larger groups; healthy or sick; and at all stages of the life cycle."[6]

Some titles need to be clarified at this point: *dietitian*; *registered dietitian*; *registered dietitian nutritionist*; *nutritionist*; *licensed dietitian*; *dietetic technician, registered*; and *nutrition and dietetics technician, registered* (**Figure 2–2**). The title of dietitian usually implies a registered dietitian (RD or RDN). There is no difference between an RD and an RDN. For the sake of simplicity, the acronym RDN will be used throughout this book. An RDN has completed

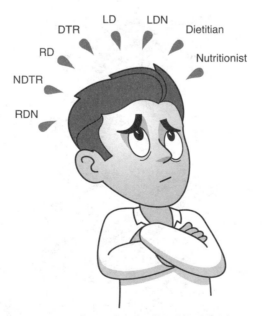

FIGURE 2–2 Titles used in the dietetics profession.

the required academic training and supervised practice program (described in Chapters 5 and 6) and has successfully passed the national credentialing exam. There are no such requirements for the use of the title "nutritionist"; the term has no standards of education or training. This means that anyone can use the title nutritionist with little or no training in the field—and many do. A few states restrict the use of these titles unless the person has completed a certain amount of education and training.[7]

Many states have regulatory laws that either require or permit dietitians to be licensed. A licensed dietitian or licensed dietitian/nutritionist (LD or LDN) is a person who has been licensed by a state to ensure competence. State requirements for licensure are frequently met through the same education, training, and national exam required for RDNs.[7]

Registered dietitian nutritionist (RDN) is a nationally recognized title for a nutrition expert. This title reflects the high level of entry-level education and training and the continuing education required to achieve and maintain RDN status. In addition, some RDNs have achieved additional certification in specialized areas of practice, such as pediatric nutrition (CSP, Board Certified Specialist in Pediatric Nutrition), renal nutrition (CSR, Board Certified Specialist in Renal Nutrition), sports nutrition (CSSD, Board Certified Specialist in Sports Dietetics), gerontologic nutrition (CSG, Board Certified Specialist in Gerontological Nutrition), and oncology nutrition (CSO, Board Certified Specialist in Oncology Nutrition).[7]

The title *dietetic technician, registered* (DTR) or *nutrition and dietetics technician, registered* (NDTR), like dietitian, implies that the person is a registered dietetic technician or nutrition and dietetics technician. There is no difference between a DTR and an NDTR. For the sake of simplicity, the acronym NDTR will be used throughout this book (**Figure 2–3**). NDTRs are

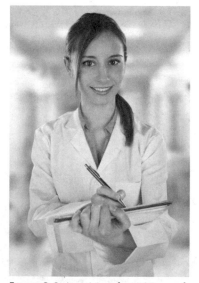

FIGURE 2–3 A registered nutrition and dietetics technician (NDTR) at work.
© BONNINSTUDIO/ Shutterstock

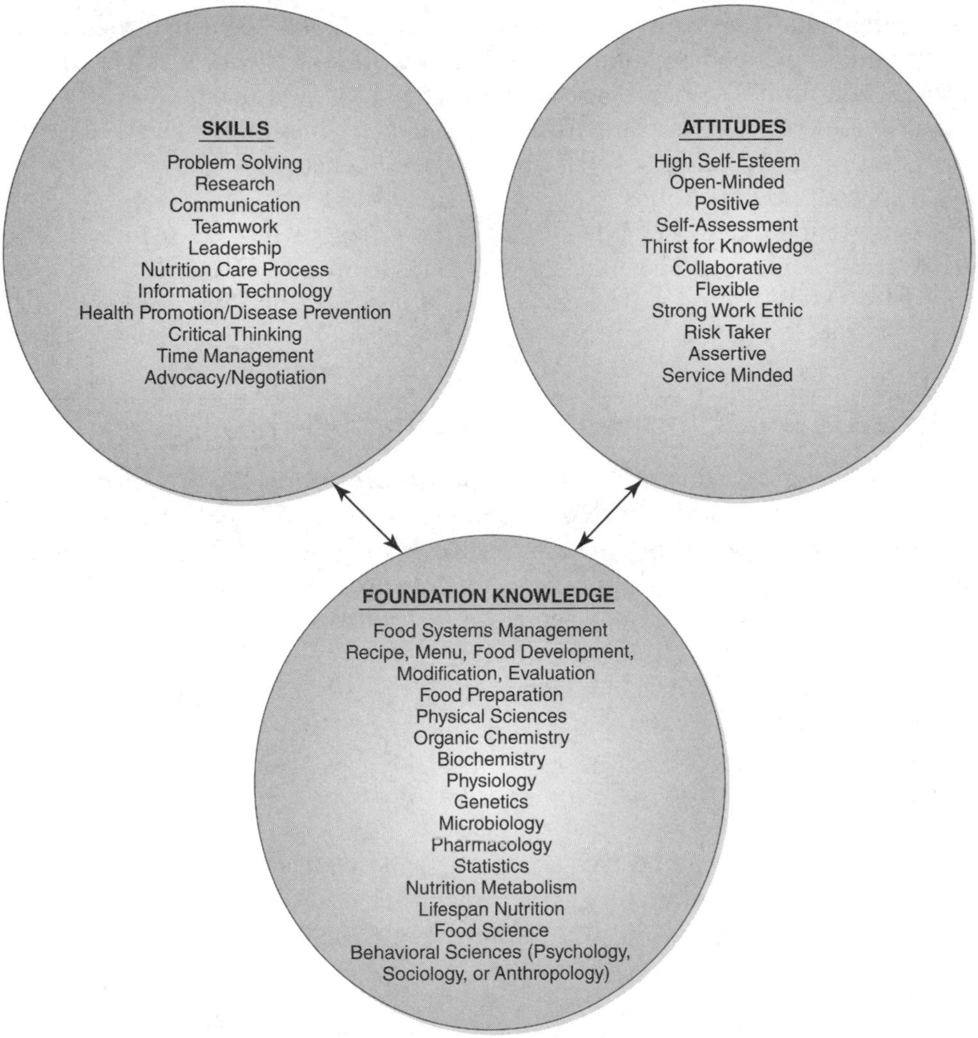

SKILLS

Problem Solving
Research
Communication
Teamwork
Leadership
Nutrition Care Process
Information Technology
Health Promotion/Disease Prevention
Critical Thinking
Time Management
Advocacy/Negotiation

ATTITUDES

High Self-Esteem
Open-Minded
Positive
Self-Assessment
Thirst for Knowledge
Collaborative
Flexible
Strong Work Ethic
Risk Taker
Assertive
Service Minded

FOUNDATION KNOWLEDGE

Food Systems Management
Recipe, Menu, Food Development,
Modification, Evaluation
Food Preparation
Physical Sciences
Organic Chemistry
Biochemistry
Physiology
Genetics
Microbiology
Pharmacology
Statistics
Nutrition Metabolism
Lifespan Nutrition
Food Science
Behavioral Sciences (Psychology,
Sociology, or Anthropology)

FIGURE 2–4 Model for dietetic practice.

trained in food and nutrition and are an integral part of healthcare and food-service management teams. Like RDNs, NDTRs must complete an academic program and a supervised practice experience and must pass a national written exam in order to use the title.[7]

Dietetic practice is based on the application of principles derived from the integration of knowledge from many disciplines. Successful dietetic practitioners then apply skills and attitudes to translate this knowledge in order to achieve and maintain the health of people. **Figure 2–4** is a graphic depiction of the knowledge areas, skills, and attitudes essential for successful dietetic practice.

Who Are Dietitians?

A recent survey, which included a sample of 9,058 members of the Academy of Nutrition and Dietetics, found that 95% of dietetic practitioners are female, with a median age of 46. The field is predominantly white; 9% of respondents indicated a race other than white, and 4% identified themselves as Hispanic. The median number of years of work experience was 16. Almost all RDNs hold bachelor's degrees, with 47% having a master's degree and 4% a doctorate. Sixty-seven percent of RDNs are members of the Academy of Nutrition and Dietetics, 44% have a state license, and 21% hold one or more specialty certifications.[3]

Thirty-nine percent of NDTRs hold a bachelor's degree or higher, and 40% are members of the Academy of Nutrition and Dietetics. Five percent of NDTRs hold a state license, and 11% hold one or more specialty certifications.[3]

Where Do Dietitians Work, and What Do They Do?

Dietitians seem to work everywhere and do everything. More specifically, the professional association's 2013 Compensation and Benefit Survey found that the most common employment setting is the hospital: 24% of dietitians and 33% of NDTRs work in a hospital setting. Ten percent of RDNs and 27% of NDTRs work in an extended-care facility, 12% of RDNs and 1% of NDTRs work in a clinic or ambulatory care center, and 7% of RDNs and 8% of NDTRs work in a community or public health program. The remaining practitioners work in a wide variety of other settings (**Figure 2–5**). Eight percent are self-employed (primarily RDNs), 38% work for a nonprofit firm, 30% work for a for-profit company, and 19% work for the government.[3]

Dietetic practice can be divided into seven key areas: clinical—acute care/inpatient, clinical—ambulatory care, clinical—long-term care, food and nutrition management, community, consultation and business, and education and

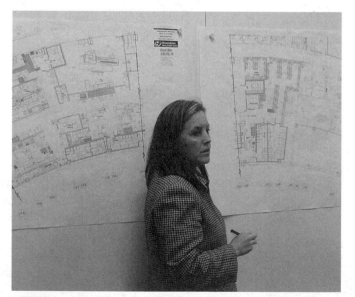

FIGURE 2–5 A dietitian who works for a foodservice facility design company.
Courtesy of Christine Guyott, RD

TABLE 2–1

Percentage of Dietitians in the Seven Practice Areas in the Field of Dietetics

Practice Area	RDNs	NDTRs
Clinical nutrition—acute care/inpatient	32%	44%
Clinical nutrition—ambulatory care	17%	1%
Clinical nutrition—long-term care	8%	13%
Food and nutrition management	12%	19%
Community	11%	11%
Consultation and business	8%	2%
Education and research	6%	2%

NDTRs, nutrition and dietetics technician, registered; RDNs, registered dietitian nutritionist.
Data from: Academy of Nutrition and Dietetics. *2013 Compensation and Benefits Survey of the Dietetics Profession*. Chicago: Academy of Nutrition and Dietetics; 2014.

research. Within these seven areas, 40 different job titles account for 80% of all dietetic employment.[8] The percentage breakdown for those working in these seven practice areas is shown in **Table 2–1**.

The following are the most commonly held position titles in dietetic practice (note that the percentages of the top 12 positions for RDNs and the top 5 for NDTRs are given in parentheses):

Clinical—Acute Care/Inpatient
Dietetic technician, clinical (42%)
Clinical dietitian (16%)
Clinical dietitian, specialist—cardiac
Clinical dietitian, specialist—diabetes
Clinical dietitian, specialist—oncology
Clinical dietitian, specialist—renal
Clinical dietitian, specialist—other
Pediatric/neonatal dietitian (3%)
Nutrition support dietitian (3%)

Clinical—Ambulatory Care
Outpatient dietitian, general (4%)
Outpatient dietitian, specialist—cardiac rehabilitation
Outpatient dietitian, specialist—diabetes (4%)
Outpatient dietitian, specialist—pediatrics
Outpatient dietitian, specialist—renal (3%)
Outpatient dietitian, specialist—weight management
Outpatient dietitian, specialist—other
Home-care dietitian

Clinical—Long-Term Care
Clinical dietitian, long-term care (8%)
Dietetic technician, long-term care (12%)

Food and Nutrition Management
Executive-level professional
Administrative dietitian—patient care
Assistant director of foodservices
Clinical nutrition manager (3%)
Director of food and nutrition services (5% of RDNs and 6% of NDTRs)
School foodservice director
Dietetic technician, foodservice management (10%)

Community
Women, Infants, and Children (WIC) nutritionist (6% of RDNs and 8% of NDTRs)
Cooperative extension educator/specialist
Corrections dietitian
Public health nutritionist (3%)
School/child care nutritionist
Nutrition coordinator for Head Start program
Nutritionist for food bank or assistance program

Consultation and Business
Private practice dietitian—patient/client nutrition care (2%)
Consultant—communications
Sales representative
Consultant—community and/or corporate programs
Public relations and/or marketing professional
Corporate account manager
Corporate dietitian
Director of nutrition
Manager of nutrition communications
Research and development nutritionist

Education and Research
Instructor/lecturer
Assistant or associate professor
Chair, Department of Nutrition and Food Science
Clinical research dietitian
Administrator, higher education
Didactic program director
Dietetic internship director
Professor[3]

In summary, most RDNs are found in the following settings:

- **Hospitals, health maintenance organizations (HMOs), and other health-care facilities.** RDNs educate patients about nutrition and administer medical nutrition therapy (MNT) as part of the healthcare team. They also manage the foodservice operation, where they oversee everything from food purchasing and preparation to managing the staff (**Figure 2–6**).

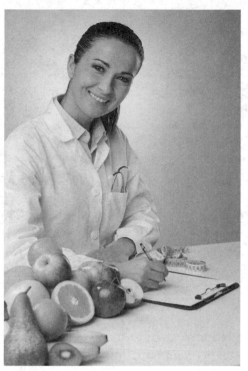

FIGURE 2–6 A clinical dietitian.
© Stock-Asso/Shutterstock

- **Schools, day care centers, and correctional facilities.** RDNs manage the foodservice operations, including planning menus, purchasing food, supervising preparation, and directing the staff (**Figure 2–7**).
- **Sports nutrition and corporate wellness programs.** RDNs educate clients about the connections among food, fitness, and health (**Figure 2–8**).

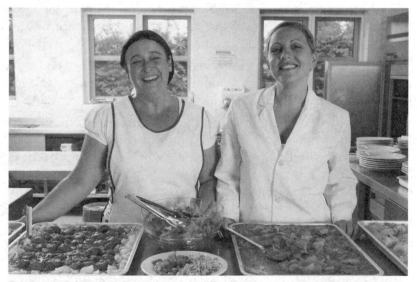

FIGURE 2–7 A dietitian who works in school foodservice and one of her employees.
© Monkey Business Images/Shutterstock

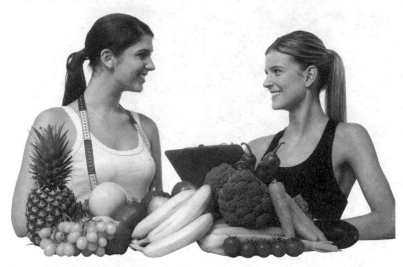

FIGURE 2–8 Two dietitians who work in sports nutrition.
© stockyimages/Shutterstock

- **Food- and nutrition-related businesses and industries.** RDNs work in communications, consumer affairs, public relations, marketing, and product development.
- **Private practice.** RDNs work under contract with healthcare or food companies or in their own business. RDNs provide services to restaurant and foodservice managers, food vendors and distributors, athletes, nursing home residents, and company employees.
- **Community and public health settings.** RDNs teach, monitor, advise, and help the public to improve their quality of life through the promotion of healthy eating habits.
- **Universities and medical centers.** RDNs teach physicians, nurses, dietetics students and interns, and others the science of food and nutrition.
- **Research facilities.** RDNs direct and collaborate on experimental research to answer critical questions at food and pharmaceutical companies, universities, and hospitals.[9]

NDTRs may also be found working independently or in teams with RDNs in a variety of work settings, including health care, business and industry, public health, foodservice, and research. NDTRs most commonly work in:

- **Hospitals, HMOs, clinics, nursing homes, retirement centers, hospices, home healthcare agencies, and research facilities.** NDTRs treat and prevent disease and administer MNT as an important part of the healthcare team.
- **Schools, day care centers, correctional facilities, restaurants, healthcare facilities, corporations, and hospitals.** NDTRs manage foodservice operations, including food purchasing and preparation, supervising employees, and teaching nutrition classes (**Figure 2–9**).
- **WIC programs, public health agencies, Meals on Wheels, and community health programs.** NDTRs develop and teach nutrition classes for the public.

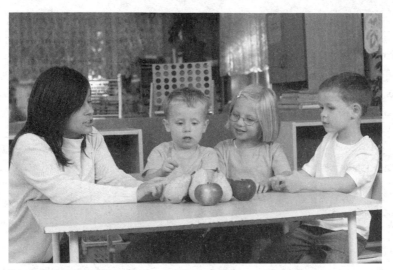

FIGURE 2–9 An NDTR teaching a nutrition class for preschoolers.
© matka_Wariatka/Shutterstock

- **Health clubs, weight-management clinics, and community wellness centers.** NDTRs educate clients about the connections among food, fitness, and health.
- **Food companies, contract food management companies, food vendors, and food distribution companies.** NDTRs develop menus, oversee foodservice sanitation and food safety, and prepare food labeling information and nutrient analysis.[9]

What Is the Salary Range for RDNs and NDTRs?

As is true for most professions, the salary range and fees charged vary by region of the country, employment setting, scope of responsibility, and supply and demand for RDNs. According to the professional association's 2013 Compensation and Benefits Survey, the median annual income in the United States for dietitians who have been working at least 1 year is $61,000, and for NDTRs who have been working in a position for at least 1 year, it is $40,000.[3] The U.S. Bureau of Labor Statistics 2014 data found the median salary for RDNs was $57,000 and the median salary for NDTRs was $26,000. It is unclear why these discrepancies exist.

The statistics generated by the survey from the Academy of Nutrition and Dietetics show that the dietitian's salary increases as the number of years in the field increases, as the number of years in the position increases, as higher graduate degrees are held, as the level and scope of responsibility increase, as the size of the budget that is managed increases, as the size of the employing organization increases, and as the number of people being supervised increases.[3]

Two other factors have an influence on salary—the area of practice and the area of the country. The highest paying practice areas are food and nutrition management, consultation and business, and education and research.

The lowest paying areas are in clinical and community nutrition practice. According to the Bureau of Labor Statistics, the highest salaries were found in California, Maryland, Nevada, Connecticut, and New Jersey. The top-paying metropolitan areas were all in California:

- San Francisco Bay Area
- Oakland
- Vallejo
- Salinas

In addition to pay, fringe benefits are an important employment consideration. When compared with benefits of other professional technical employees in private industry, dietetic professionals' benefits are very favorable. The percentage of practitioners offered various benefits is shown in Table 2–2.

TABLE 2–2

Benefits Offered to Dietetics Professionals

Benefit	% of Employers Offering Benefit
Paid vacation, personal time off	82
Paid holidays	72
Paid sick days	68
Medical insurance, high deductible	54
Medical insurance, lower deductible	66
Dental insurance or group plan	81
Prescription drug benefit	73
Vision insurance or group plan	75
Life insurance	78
Disability insurance (long- and/or short-term)	74
Defined contribution retirement plan	72
Defined benefit retirement plan (pension)	25
Stock options	8
Profit sharing	8
Funding for professional development	55
Professional society dues	20
College tuition assistance	46
Employee assistance or wellness program	53
Comptime or flextime	32
Fitness benefit	42
Extended and/or paid parental leave	40
On-site child care or allowance	10
Telecommuting	13

Data from: Academy of Nutrition and Dietetics. *2013 Compensation and Benefits Survey of the Dietetics Profession.* Chicago: Academy of Nutrition and Dietetics; 2014.

Specialty Areas and New Employment Opportunities

The dietetic profession is committed to helping people enjoy healthy lives. Therefore, five critical health areas confronting Americans have become priorities for the dietetics profession: (1) obesity and overweight, (2) aging, (3) complementary care and dietary supplements, (4) safe and nutritious food supply, and (5) human genome and genetics. Opportunities abound in these areas, as they do in the less traditional dietetic careers.[9]

As mentioned earlier, dietitians can be found working most anywhere. Consider the following nutrition-related employment opportunities that have not been mentioned previously:

Attorney
Author
Chef (**Figure 2–10**)
Educational representative for business
Extension service 4-H coordinator
Extension service home advisor
Food advertising consultant
Food analyst/technologist
Food broker
Food editor
Food journalist
Food photography specialist
Food quality assurance specialist
Food research and marketing specialist
Food science educator
Food scientist
Foodservice administrator for airline or cruise line

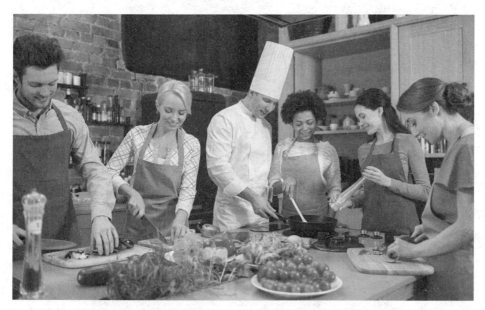

FIGURE 2–10 A dietitian who is a chef teaching a healthy cooking class.
© Syda Productions/Shutterstock

Foodservice equipment specialist
Food stylist
Freelance writer
Home economist for food, equipment, or utility business
Job listing and placement service executive
Marketing specialist for a food or nutrition company
Media spokesperson
Motivational speaker
Peace Corps representative
Product development researcher
Publisher
Rehabilitation consultant
Research chemist (**Figure 2–11**)
Restaurant owner
Taste panel coordinator
Test kitchen scientist

This list is by no means exhaustive, but it shows the breadth of opportunities available to someone who has training in food and nutrition. The educational requirements for these positions vary from some college work to an advanced degree. Many do not require any credential, but some do. Some require additional training and/or education other than an advanced degree.

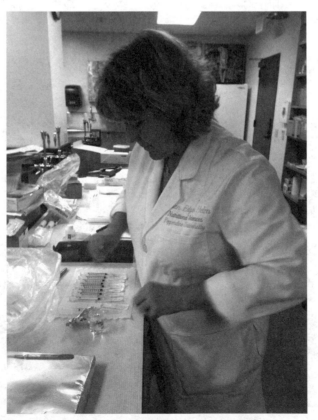

FIGURE 2–11 A dietitian/professor conducting research.
Courtesy of Susan Helm, PhD, RDN, Pepperdine University

What Are Some of the Issues Facing Dietetic Practice?

This is an exciting time to be a nutrition professional. According to the U.S. Bureau of Labor Statistics, the employment of nutritionist dietitians is projected to grow 21% from 2012 to 2022. This is faster than the average of all occupations. The role of food in preventing and treating diseases, such as diabetes and heart disease, is now well known. The understanding that lifestyle choices, such as diet and exercise, can make a dramatic difference in quality of life is now widespread. People are eager for information that can give them an edge in competitive sports, improve their appearance, make them feel better, and help them live longer, more productive lives. The knowledge that what we eat can dramatically affect our health will create a demand for those who can provide this information. Everybody needs us! Obesity is a worldwide health issue. A government-sponsored research study recently showed that the annual healthcare cost of obesity in the United States has doubled in less than a decade and may be as high as $147 billion a year.[10] Many people do not even know how to cook. In addition, the demand for quality control and reliability in the food industry is increasing.

Job growth in health care continues to be strong. The health-related professions have not suffered from the recent recession because of the aging of the U.S. population and increases in the number and type of available treatments. According to one expert, "While fast-food and customer-service may churn out a greater total volume of new jobs, those in health care are almost as plentiful and offer better pay, prospects, and benefits, plus the stability of a nearly recession-proof industry."[11] Over the next several years, job growth in health care is expected to be twice that of other industries. A number of factors account for this growth. The "graying of America" will create the need for more specialized medical care, home health care, and geriatric specialists. The increasing focus on wellness and preventive medicine by HMOs and by the public at large has also contributed to the expansion of the healthcare field.

The three fastest-growing career fields are health care, computers, and education. Dietetic practitioners are widely employed in each of these fields. Jobs that require a bachelor's degree or higher will grow at a rate almost double that of jobs that require only a high school diploma. Specific to the area of dietetics and nutrition, job growth will result from an increasing emphasis on disease prevention through improved dietary habits. The growing aging population will boost demand for nutritional counseling in hospitals, residential care facilities, schools, prisons, community health programs, and home healthcare agencies. The public's growing interest in nutrition, health education, and a prudent lifestyle will increase demand, especially in foodservice management. In addition, the increased prevalence and awareness of obesity and diabetes have resulted in Medicare coverage being expanded to include medical nutrition therapy for renal and diabetic patients. Dietitians specializing in these fields will benefit from this coverage.

The areas predicted to experience the fastest growth in job opportunities for dietetic practitioners are outpatient care facilities, physician offices, and foodservice management. Dietitians with specialized training, advanced degrees, and certifications beyond their state's minimum requirements will enjoy the best job opportunities. Those specializing in renal disease, diabetes, or gerontology will benefit from the growing number of people with diabetes and the aging of the population.

However, there may be some clouds on the otherwise rosy horizon of the healthcare industry. Cost-containment measures, such as budget cutting, downsizing, realignments, outsourcing, and mergers, may affect growth. Many predict that funding for Medicare programs will be reduced, forcing Medicare patients to pay for some home-care costs themselves. However, government surveys of job prospects indicate that healthcare reform will not shrink the workforce.

Negative factors specifically affecting job opportunities in dietetics and nutrition include the fact that some employers are substituting lower-paid workers to do nutrition-related work. Also, the demand for nutritional counseling is related to the patients' ability to pay, either out-of-pocket or through insurance reimbursement. Although the extent of insurance coverage for nutrition services has increased, it still varies widely. Hospitals and nursing care facilities still continue to employ large numbers of dietitians and dietetic technicians, but they also continue to contract with outside firms to run the foodservice operation and move medical nutrition therapy to outpatient departments.

Although dietetic practitioners are regarded as experts in nutrition, there is still some lack of recognition from the public. The American public has increased its knowledge and understanding of foods and nutrition, but misinformation still abounds. Popular magazines are full of attention-grabbing, but inaccurate, advice. Health food stores promote the sale of supposedly "super nutrients" to the tune of billions of dollars a year. Many people lack the educational background to discern a good study from a poor one. Many believe that if it's in print, it must be true.

A Brief Introduction to the Professional Association

The Academy of Nutrition and Dietetics is the oldest and most prominent professional organization for dietitians (it is discussed at length in Chapter 8). Among the most important functions of the Academy is the development of Standards of Practice and Standards of Professional Performance, outlining a dietetic practitioner's responsibilities for providing quality nutritional care. The standards provide individual practitioners with a systematic plan for implementing, evaluating, and adjusting performance in any area of practice.[9] See Chapter 7 for a discussion of the standards.

Because of the increasingly specialized nature of dietetic practice, the leadership of the Academy developed board certification in some specialty areas and Dietetic Practice Groups (DPGs). DPGs provide a way for members of the association to network and share specialized information within their area or areas of interest and practice. Currently, the Academy of Nutrition and Dietetics supports 26 DPGs and 30 subunits of these DPGs, which are described in Chapter 8 (**Figure 2–12**).

Another important function of the Academy is its recognition of excellence in practice through awards given annually by the national organization

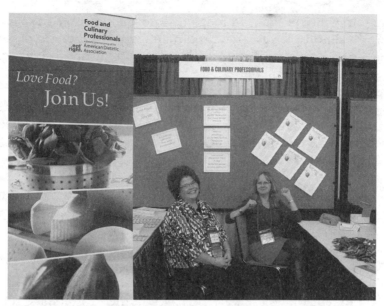

FIGURE 2–12 The Food and Culinary Professionals Dietetic Practice Group's booth at the Food and Nutrition Conference and Exposition.
Courtesy of the Academy of Nutrition and Dietetics

and by its affiliated state associations.[9] See Chapter 8 for a list and description of these awards.

Summary

The horizon leans forward
Offering you space
To place new steps of change

—Excerpt from "On the Pulse of Morning," 1993
presidential inaugural poem by Maya Angelou[12]

The scope of dietetic practice is almost limitless. The creation of new, exciting positions that make use of food and nutrition education and training will continue as long as members of the profession have the imagination and determination to succeed.

"The world is happier, healthier, [and] better off because of the work you do," proclaimed Rabbi Harold S. Kushner to the dietetic professionals gathered at a recent dietetic association national conference.[13] The work of dietetics is considered a profession because it requires a specialized body of knowledge; because members render specialized services to society; because their obligations to serve override personal considerations; and because members consider competence, honor, continuing education, research, and sharing of knowledge for the common good to be necessary.

Dietetic practice encompasses nutrition therapy, the food industry, health promotion/disease prevention, foodservice systems, entrepreneurship, and education. Drawing on their training and knowledge in the fields of science, leadership, technology, research, and management, dietetic professionals communicate and collaborate to provide food and nutrition services for individuals, groups, and communities.

Dietetic practitioners work in private practice or in a hospital, with patients referred by physicians for help in implementing necessary nutritional modifications. Dietetic practitioners serve as consultants in corporate wellness programs, weight-loss programs, and eating disorder clinics. Professional athletes and athletic teams often have full-time dietitians on their training staff.

Dietetic practitioners are also involved in scientific research and education. Increasing numbers of dietitians have careers in sales, marketing, and public relations for the food industry, pharmaceutical and computer companies, and equipment manufacturers. They are involved in many areas of community work, especially with pregnant women, women with infants and young children, and the elderly.

Dietetic practitioners are particularly qualified to manage foodservice operations in hospitals, nursing homes, colleges and universities, public schools, commercial restaurants, correctional facilities, catering operations, airline commissaries, and community programs. Interest is growing in combining nutrition credentials with other degrees, such as those in business, law, nursing, physical fitness, and the culinary arts.

The Academy of Nutrition and Dietetics has developed DPGs to enable members to network and increase their knowledge within their particular area of practice. The Academy also offers annual awards for excellence in specific areas of practice and develops and promotes standards of practice that outline a dietetic practitioner's responsibilities for providing quality nutritional care.

Societal needs are best served by having a population that is adequately nourished. Dietetics serves people by offering correct and current information so that individuals can make their own choices. The education, training, and knowledge of dietitians make them uniquely qualified to help individuals and society meet their nutritional needs.

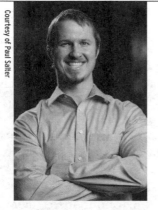

Courtesy of Paul Salter

Profile of a Professional

Paul Salter, MS, RD, LD, CSCS

Nutrition Editor
Bodybuilding.com

Sports Nutrition Consultant
Renaissance Periodization, Boise, Idaho

Education:
BS in Dietetics, University of Maryland, College Park, Maryland
Dietetic Internship, Beaumont Health Systems, Royal Oak, Michigan
MS in Exercise and Nutrition Sciences, University of Tampa, Tampa, Florida

How did you first hear about dietetics and decide to become a Registered Dietitian?
I learned of the Registered Dietitian (RD) credential during my freshman year of college while taking a general education requirement: Elements of Nutrition (Nutrition 101). This class sparked an interest that had always existed, but never fully blossomed. The professor of my class played a prominent role as she outlined the various paths I could take with the RD credential.

What was your route to registration?
I completed my dietetic internship following graduation with a Bachelor's of Science in dietetics. I applied for the Fall Dietetic Internship match and was fortunate enough to begin my internship approximately 7 months after graduating.

At what college or university did you receive your entry-level education?
I completed my BS in Dietetics from the University of Maryland in May 2013. I then completed my Dietetic Internship at Beaumont Health Systems in Royal Oak, Michigan (January–August 2014), with a concentration in medical nutrition therapy. I completed a 12-month intensive master's program at the University of Tampa and earned a Master's of Science in Exercise and Nutrition Sciences.

Where did you complete your supervised practice experience?
I completed my Dietetic Internship at Beaumont Health Systems in Royal Oak, Michigan (January–August 2014), with a concentration in medical nutrition therapy.

Do you have advanced degree(s)? If so, in what and from where?
I have an MS in Exercise and Nutrition Sciences from the University of Tampa. I am also a Certified Strength and Conditioning Specialist (CSCS) through the National Strength and Conditioning Association (NSCA).

How are you involved professionally?
I am consistently learning via online quizzes and attending conferences for both the Academy of Nutrition and Dietetics (AND) and the NSCA. I have moved six times in the past 3 years (pursuing my dreams) but have been fortunate enough to deliver online presentations and serve as a guest speaker for students interested in sports nutrition and dietetics. I also stay active via online communities to help answer questions for those interested in the nutrition field.

What honors or awards have you received?
- Outstanding Graduate Student, University of Tampa, May 2015
- Campus Recreation Services (University of Maryland) Student Employee Scholarship, Spring 2015
- Men's Novice Lightweight and Overall Champion, National Gym Association, Annapolis Cup, June 2012

Briefly describe your career path in dietetics. What are you doing now?
I have been very fortunate to have had the opportunity to complete various experiences in the field of sports nutrition. They're best summed up in a list:

- Sports Nutrition Intern, George Mason University, Fairfax, Virginia: Worked with sports dietitian; shadowed sessions, completed projects, discussed current research.
- St. Vincent's Sports Performance Center, National Football League (NFL) Combine Preparation Program, Indianapolis, Indiana: Worked alongside sports dietitian, strength coaches, sport psychologists, and medical staff to best prepare athletes for NFL Combine. Participated in one-on-one counseling, group sessions, menu planning, meal planning, and other various forms of education.
- Gatorade Sports Nutrition Immersion Program (SNIP), University of North Carolina (UNC), Chapel Hill, North Carolina: I was one of six students in the nation selected for this program. I had the opportunity to work alongside two sports dietitians at UNC for a 5-month period while being paid by Gatorade.
  - Worked directly with football team to adequately fuel and hydrate student-athletes throughout training camp.

- ◦ Conducted body composition tests (BodPod), nutrition screenings, supplement reviews, and hydration tests (urine specific gravity).
- ◦ Collaborated with dietitians to lead grocery store and dining hall tours for student-athletes on various teams.
- ◦ Managed athletics department's Gatorade budget and carried out nutrition product distribution.
- ◦ Provided educational materials to student-athletes and coaches utilizing print materials, presentations, and new media.
- ◦ Contributed to the training and development of other interns within the Sports Nutrition Department.
- Beaumont Health Systems Dietetic Internship, Royal Oak, Michigan
- IMG Academy, full-time Nutrition Coach/Sports Dietitian:
  - ◦ Deliver one-on-one and group sessions for full-time student-athletes, camp athletes, professional athletes, and corporate partners accordingly to a broad client base ranging from youth to elite athletes across a range of sports, cultures, and countries.
  - ◦ Educate, develop, and execute nutritional supplement strategies for professional athletes at IMG Academy.
  - ◦ Oversee IMG Academy professional athlete nutritional supplement program, including education, development, preparation, delivery, inventory, and documentation.
  - ◦ Collaborate with food and beverage staff, coaches, and entire performance team to optimally fuel student-athletes.
  - ◦ Deliver in-service education sessions to campus staff.

I have had several diverse experiences in the field of sports nutrition and am forever thankful for each and every experience and every contact I made.

I currently serve as the Nutrition Editor for Bodybuilding.com, where I write, edit, and oversee all nutrition-related articles and content published on the website. I also consult with Renaissance Periodization, where I work one-on-one (online) with clients and athletes of various ages, sports, and goals to help them fuel for optimal health, body composition, and performance.

What excites you about dietetics and the future of our profession?
The field of nutrition is gaining more respect each and every day, specifically within the realm of sports nutrition. When I first became interested, roughly 5 years ago, there were a mere 19 full-time sports dietitians across both the collegiate and professional level. Today, there are well over 100 in addition to countless part-time positions, graduate assistant positions, and internships. Athletic performance has seen a great improvement when exposed to the work of a talented sports dietitian, and I am excited to see how far we can push human performance through proper fueling in the years to come.

How is teamwork important to you in your position? How have you been involved in team projects?
The performance team is composed of the sports dietitian(s), strength coaches, sports psychologists, medical staff, and athletic trainers. I was fortunate enough to have each area of expertise under one roof during my time at IMG. Having countless opportunities to share information about athletes with each professional helped all of us to do our jobs better because we were aware of every factor affecting the athlete—injuries, stress, progress, habits, etc. Teamwork is invaluable as it provides numerous pairs of eyes on a similar situation, which allows multiple ideas to be combined to generate the best process and outcome.

What words of wisdom do you have for future dietetics professionals?
Absolutely follow your dreams, wherever they may take you. Do not worry about money, travel, etc., because happiness is the true measure of success, and if you love what you do, finances and travel should not matter.

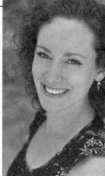

Profile of a Professional

Whitney Ellersick, MS, RDN

Assistant Director, Nutrition Services Department
Portland Public Schools, Portland, Oregon

Education:
BS in Clinical Nutrition, University of California, Davis, California
Dietetic Internship, Oregon Health and Science University, Portland, Oregon
MS in Clinical Nutrition, Oregon Health and Science University, Portland, Oregon

How did you first hear about dietetics and decide to become a Registered Dietitian?
I first had an interest in nutrition when I was in the fifth grade and a teacher introduced us to nutrition concepts of how various foods fuel our bodies and play a role in our overall health. It was also around this time that my mom took an interest in cooking healthier options for our family in order to help my dad reduce his cholesterol levels. I loved and excelled in the sciences, so I knew that this was the area for me.

What was your route to registration?
I completed my internship and MS in Clinical Nutrition at Oregon Health and Science University in Portland, Oregon.

Where did you complete your supervised practice experience?
I completed my supervised practice in my internship at Oregon Health and Science University. The majority of my supervised practice was at the Portland Veterans Affairs Medical Center but also included time at the Salud Women, Infants and Children (WIC) Program, Western Culinary Institute, and Shriners Children's Hospital.

Do you have advanced degree(s)? If so, in what and from where?
I graduated with my MS in Clinical Nutrition from Oregon Health and Science University. I was one of the first three students to graduate from their graduate program. The internship, supervised practice hours, and research thesis were completed within 22 months.

What are some examples of your professional involvement at the local, state, or national level at the American Dietetic Association (ADA)/Academy of Nutrition and Dietetics or other professional associations?

CIA Healthy Kids Collaborative Member: 2015–current
School Food FOCUS National Procurement Initiative Task Force: 2014–current
Oregon Academy of Nutrition and Dietetics Director of Communication and Publication
Board Member: 2013–current
Dietetic Preceptor/Mentor to distance programs, undergraduate students, and high school students: 2013–current
Medical Teams International Volunteer, Honduras: March 2010
Oregon Health and Science University Dietetic Internship Advisory Council Member: 2009–current
Oregon Health and Science University Dietetic Internship Preceptor: 2008–current
Oregon Health and Science University Dietetic Internship Guest Lecturer: 2008–current
School Nutrition Association and Oregon School Nutrition Association: 2007–current
Oregon Health and Science University Masters Curriculum Committee–Masters Handbook Sub-Committee: 2007
Commission on Accreditation for Dietetics Education (CADE), American Dietetic Association

Student Representative: 2005–2006
Student Council Advisory Committee, American Dietetic Association
Student Representative: 2005–2006
Nominations Committee within Student Council Advisory Committee: 2005–2006

What are some of the awards and honors you have received?

- 2014 Oregon Academy of Nutrition and Dietetics Recognized Young Dietitian of the Year Award
- National Outstanding Preceptor Award Nominee, June 2013
- "You Rock" Award 2013—presented by Portland Public Schools, COO CJ Sylvestor
- "30 under 30," *FoodService Director* Magazine, September 2011
- Oregon Dietetic Association Outstanding Student Award, 2005

Briefly describe your career path in dietetics. What are you doing now?
After graduating from Oregon Health and Science University (OHSU), I continued to work for my thesis mentor, Diane Stadler, PhD, RD, LD, as a research assistant at OHSU. That spring, I applied for a new management position within the Portland Public Schools Nutrition Services Department. I was offered the position and joined an amazing team. After 4 years, I was promoted to Senior Program Manager, and then in 2014, I applied for and was offered the position as Assistant Director for the department. As Assistant Director, I am responsible for leading the operations and supply chain teams for the department, which includes 85 schools and about 240 employees.

What excites you about dietetics and the future of our profession?
Dietetics is an ever-changing and evolving field. The possibilities continue to unfold for emerging professionals. Colleagues all over the country are creating new opportunities and promoting the profession in new ways, advocating for our citizens, communities, and their health.

How is teamwork important to you in your position? How have you been involved in team projects?
Teamwork is essential to our daily operations, our effectiveness as managers, and the success of our department. Communication is one of the key pieces to our teamwork, and we are always working to understand and improve in this area. Everyone must be willing to do all tasks and not be afraid to get involved and assist coworkers when needed. Creating the right teamwork culture within an organization is important to the work environment and employee satisfaction.

What words of wisdom do you have for future dietetics professionals?
I am passionate about school foodservice and absolutely love my profession. My days are never the same, and I am continuously challenged in various ways. I am able to use almost all of my knowledge and skills acquired throughout my education and my life experience. I work with amazing people to feed over 30,000 students each day, and each day, I am proud and in awe of my team for having made such a positive impact in our community. My dad told me to "keep my eyes and ears open for all opportunities," and I continued to say yes to all that I encountered; this helped me get to where I am today.

Suggested Activities

1. Dietetic Practice Groups (DPGs) are a good way to network with professionals who work in specific areas of dietetics. Visit www.eatright.org or refer to Chapter 8 of this book for a complete listing of the 26 DPGs. Choose one of the DPGs you might be interested in joining

later in your career. If possible, attend one of the meetings of this practice group at a national meeting of the Academy of Nutrition and Dietetics or at a regional meeting. Or, interview a member of the practice group to find out what the practice group does to benefit the profession and its individual members.

2. Add to the list of specialty areas of dietetic practice discussed in the chapter either by listing positions you know exist or by developing areas of practice or positions you would be interested in personally. Be creative!

3. Visit www.eatright.org to verify the accuracy of information in this chapter. Has anything changed since this chapter was written?

4. Interested in private practice? Two-thirds of Americans either run their own business or dream of being their own boss. If you are interested in starting your own private practice, visit www.morebusiness.com, click "Tips and Tools" on the main menu, and then click "6 Vital Entrepreneur Skills for a Successful Small Business." Evaluate your own personal characteristics. Do they match those considered to be important for entrepreneurial success? Explain. Are you more or less interested in private practice after completing this exercise? Explain. If your answer was "more interested," then you may want to take a look at www.inc.com/startup. This site offers many practical tips and good advice for starting your own business.

5. Interested in a career in foodservice management? Visit the website www.foodservice.com, click "JobSpot," and then click "Search Jobs." Which of them might be of interest to you in the future, or now? View a couple of the jobs to see what information is available online about these positions.

6. The salary differences for the various areas of the country may be related to the cost-of-living index in these areas. If you are unsure of what the cost-of-living index is, do an Internet search to find the cost-of-living index and its relationship to the consumer price index. Look up the cities and states listed in this chapter as having the highest and lowest salaries and compare them with the cost-of-living indexes listed for these cities on the Internet.

7. Some of the statistics and facts contained in this chapter may change as a result of economic conditions and other mitigating factors. Go to the Bureau of Labor Statistics website at www.bls.gov and research the latest information from the government on the job outlook for positions in which you have an interest. How does the information differ from that contained in the chapter?

8. Read the Code of Ethics in Chapter 7. As a future dietetic professional, what are some of the ways you could demonstrate that you have met the criteria for Standard 3 (The dietetics practitioner considers the health, safety, and welfare of the public at all times.)? Be sure that you have listed outcomes and/or goals that are specific and measurable.

9. What kinds of positions are available right now? Two companies started by dietitians provide job listings and placement services. Visit

their websites at www.jobsindietetics.com and www.nutritionjobs. com. How do the two sites differ? What positions are currently available? What area of dietetics are they in? Where are they located? What kinds of salaries are being offered?

10. What, in your opinion, should the dietetics profession do to address some of the issues facing practitioners today?

Selected Websites

- www.bls.gov—U.S. Department of Labor Bureau of Labor Statistics offers information on jobs and salaries across the United States.
- www.computrition.com—Computrition Foodservice Software Solutions sells computer software for the healthcare and hospitality industries.
- www.eatright.org—The Academy of Nutrition and Dietetics is the world's largest organization of food and nutrition professionals.
- www.helmpublishing.com—Helm Publishing provides continuing education for dietitians and nurses.
- www.inc.com—Inc. offers small business resources for the entrepreneur.
- www.jobsindietetics.com—Features jobs in dietetics and career services for professionals in dietetics, nutrition, and foodservice.
- www.morebusiness.com—Offers advice for entrepreneurs.
- www.nutritionjobs.com—Features career services for professionals in dietetics, nutrition, and foodservice.
- www.shfm-online.org—Society of Hospitality and Foodservice Management is a professional organization for those working in the corporate foodservice and workplace hospitality industries.

Suggested Readings

Crosby O, Moncarz R. The 2004–14 job outlook for college graduates. *Occupational Outlook Quarterly.* Available at: http://www.bls.gov/opub /ooq/2006/fall/art03.pdf. Accessed January 12, 2010.

Cullen LT. Now hiring! *Time* 2003;162(21):49–53.

Harnack L, French S. Fattening up on fast food. *J Am Diet Assoc.* 2003;103(10):1296–1297.

King K. *Helm Publishing: Books and Continuing Education for RDs, DTRs & RNs.* Lake Dallas, TX: Helm Publishing; Winter–Spring 2004.

Krieger E, Mantel C, Morreale S. Business and communications: career opportunities for dietitians. Presentation at ADA Food and Nutrition Conference & Expo. San Antonio, TX: October 2003.

Los Angeles Times. Menu of jobs available in the restaurant industry. *Careerbuilder.* December 7, 2003. www.careerbuilder.com.

Los Angeles Times. Restaurant workers step up to the plate: jobs covering a range of duties available in changing industry. *Careerbuilder.* December 7, 2003. www.careerbuilder.com.

McCluskey KW. Customer service in health care—dietetics professionals can take the lead. *J Am Diet Assoc.* 2003;103(10):1282.

U.S. Bureau of Labor Statistics. *Occupational Outlook Handbook.* Available at: www.bls.gov/ooh. Accessed March18, 2016.

O'Sullivan Maillet J. Dietetics in 2017: what does the future hold? *J Am Diet Assoc.* 2002;10:1404–1407.

Schofield M. Professional issues delegate's column: future dimensions. *Clin Nutr Manage.* 2003;22:14.

Smith Edge M. President's page: leading the future of dietetics. *J Am Diet Assoc.* 2003;103:420.

Smith Edge M. President's page: promote the profession and market our services: an ADA team effort. *J Am Diet Assoc.* 2003;103(10):1276.

Tactical Workgroup of the ADA House of Delegates. Performance, proficiency, and value of dietetics professional: an update. *J Am Diet Assoc.* 2003;103(10):1376–1379.

Thorpe M. Spotlight on nutrition innovators: DTRs pioneer new arenas. *J Am Diet Assoc.* 2003;103(10):1279–1280.

References

1. *Collins English Dictionary,* 6th ed. New York: HarperCollins; 2003.
2. *Mosby's Medical Dictionary,* 8th ed. Philadelphia: Elsevier; 2009.
3. Academy of Nutrition and Dietetics. *2013 Compensation and Benefits Survey of the American Dietetic Association.* Chicago: Academy of Nutrition and Dietetics; 2014.
4. Brandeis LD. *Business—A Profession.* University of Louisville, Louis D. Brandeis School of Law website. http://www.law.louisville.edu/library/collections/brandeis/node/202. Accessed April 26, 2010.
5. The American Dietetic Association Committee on Goals of Education for Dietetics. Goals of the lifetime education of the dietitian. *J Am Diet Assoc.* 1969;54:91–93.
6. Galbraith A. Excellence defined. *J Am Diet Assoc.* 1975;67:211.
7. Health professionals. Academy of Nutrition and Dietetics website. Available at: http://www.eatright.org/HealthProfessionals/. Accessed February 18, 2010.
8. American Dietetic Association. Hornick BA, ed. *Job Descriptions: Models for the Dietetics Profession.* Chicago: The American Dietetic Association; 2003.
9. Academy of Nutrition and Dietetics website. Available at: http://www.eatright.org. Accessed March 18, 2016.
10. Paddock C. Obesity healthcare costs US 147 billion dollars a year, new study. *Medical News Today.* Available at: http://www.medicalnewstoday.com/articles/158948.php. Accessed January 20, 2010.
11. Thottam J. Health kick. *Time* 2003;16221:54–57.
12. Angelou M. *On the Pulse of Morning.* New York: Random House; 1993.
13. American Dietetic Association. *Set Your Sights: Your Future in Dietetics.* Chicago: The American Dietetic Association; 1991.

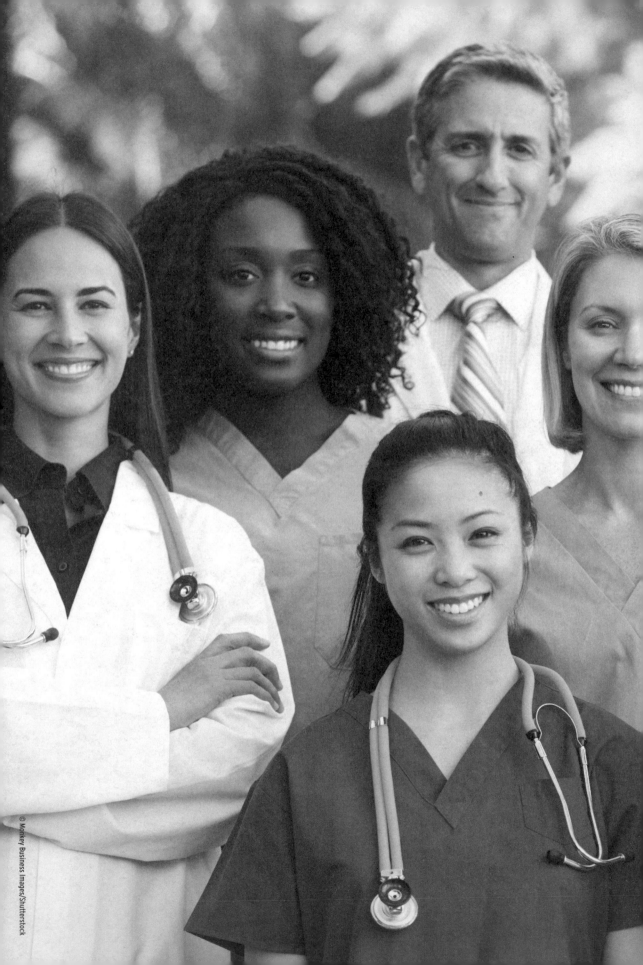

Joining Together: The Team Approach

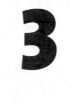

3

"My personal leadership motto is 'TEAM: Together Everyone Achieves More.'" This revelation was made by the president of the Academy of Nutrition and Dietetics, Dr. Evelyn F. Crayton, RDN, LDN, during her address at the opening session of the 2015 Food and Nutrition Conference and Expo in Nashville, Tennessee. She went on to say that an African proverb puts it this way: "If you want to go fast, go alone. If you want to go far, go together."

Have you ever heard someone say, "I prefer to work alone"? Well, they might as well forget it. Work in the twenty-first century will be done in groups and teams, specifically:

> *In all healthcare settings more work is being done by versatile and flexible multidisciplinary teams that plan, implement, and review cases. Members are valued for their ability to help the team with a "flexible eye" in making judgments and pitching in to do what needs to be done. The most valued members are those with a global view of health and proficiency in a greater number of competencies. Teams reduce costs by using fewer employees, using them synergistically, and pushing care toward lower-paid practitioners.[1]*

Because of this, it is now essential that dietetics professionals be multiskilled, cross-trained, and effective team players.

Long gone are the days of the family doctor acting alone to treat disease. Today, a career in health care is no longer limited to being either a doctor or nurse. The U.S. healthcare system is one of the most sophisticated and complex in the world. The increase in the number of older adults, shortages in the healthcare workforce, the emergence of specialized treatments that require complex technology, a new focus on preventive health care, and a better understanding of the cost benefits of a healthy workforce all create very positive prospects for anyone entering a healthcare career and serving on successful healthcare teams.

The explosion of scientific knowledge has led to a corresponding increase in the number of healthcare professions that require specialized knowledge and skills. The term *allied health* is used to describe a cluster of roles in the healthcare system that assist, facilitate, and complement the work of physicians, nurses, and pharmacists. The American Society of Allied Health Professions lists more than 100 different health service careers.[2] For example, the data acquired by laboratory technicians play a crucial role in the detection, diagnosis, and treatment of disease. The medical records administrator collects, analyzes, and manages information that steers the healthcare industry. The rehabilitation process for a patient often requires the combined efforts of physical therapists, medical social workers, occupational therapists, speech therapists, and dietitians. The hospital pharmacist works with nurses, doctors, and dietitians to provide quality patient care. These specialty areas free highly skilled medical practitioners—physicians, nurses, and pharmacists—to perform the tasks they alone are qualified to do.

In one report, a healthcare team was composed of geriatric, infectious disease, heart, and cancer physician specialists; nurses at various levels of specialization and care; physical, occupational, speech, and respiratory therapists; a dietitian; a chaplain; and a social worker. The tightly coordinated diagnosis and care by this 14-member team saved the patient's life. At the same time, each of the members of this team served on other teams with different memberships to provide care and rehabilitation to other patients. Their ability to work together on teams was the key to their success.[3]

The team approach has been used successfully in the treatment of adolescents with eating disorders. One pediatric eating disorders team might include a physician who specializes in treating the malnutrition of eating disorders and who is trained in adolescent medicine, a registered dietitian trained in adolescent medicine, a nurse, a mental health professional such as a psychiatrist or psychologist, a licensed social worker, a licensed counselor, and an advanced practice nurse.[4]

The History of the Healthcare Team Concept

The concept of the healthcare team emerged after World War II, a period of increased social awareness and higher healthcare expectations. Disabled veterans returning from the war required more than traditional medical treatment for their physical disabilities. They also needed assistance in returning to the community as socially and economically useful citizens. This led to a trend toward sharing responsibilities with other professionals that had formerly been the sole purview of the physician and/or nurse. This trend has had a major impact on the quality, costs, organization, and delivery of health care.

What Makes a Group a Team?

A **group** may be very simply defined as two or more individuals interacting with each other in such a manner that each person influences and is influenced by each other person. A group is not a team. A **team** is a small number of people with complementary skills who are committed to a common purpose, performance goals, and approach for which they hold themselves mutually accountable.[5] Two important characteristics distinguish a team from a group: (1) a team produces specific results for which the team is *collectively* responsible, and (2) a team possesses *super-consciousness* of being a team, an awareness of needing each other.[6]

Teamwork

Teamwork is the close, cooperative effort of several people to use their special skills and knowledge to meet the needs of the client/patient more efficiently, completely, competently, and considerately than would be possible by individual, independent action. An important, but often forgotten, member of the team is the client/patient.

Educating and including the client/patient in the team communication process are critically important. Because the ultimate responsibility for client/patient care rests with the physician, it is the physician who assumes the leadership role on most healthcare teams. Other members of the team vary, depending on the needs of the client/patient. A chart of possible members of a healthcare team for a patient with lung cancer is shown in **Figure 3–1**.

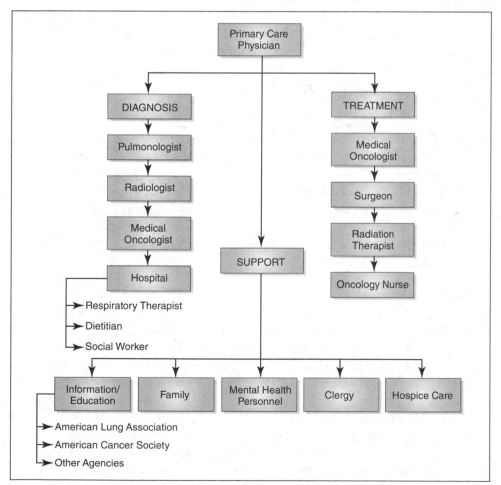

FIGURE 3–1 An organization chart showing possible members of a healthcare team for a patient with lung cancer.

To function effectively, the members of healthcare teams must be able to differentiate between roles that are unique to each discipline and roles that are shared. Team members function independently when they have unique competencies, knowledge, and experiences. **Delegated functioning** occurs when the team has varying levels and types of training.

Collaborative functioning is used when an overlap in competencies allows for a common base for judgment and decision making.

A clinical dietitian doing a patient discharge diet instruction is functioning independently. A delegated function for this same dietitian would be the implementation of a physician-prescribed diet order. An example of a collaborative, multidisciplinary approach would be the implementation of a weight-control program involving a physician, a dietitian, an exercise physiologist, a laboratory technician, and a psychologist. Diseases that have systemic effects are natural candidates for the collaborative, multidisciplinary team approach. For example, care for patients with diabetes often involves a primary care physician, an endocrinologist, a dietitian, a nurse/nurse practitioner, an ophthalmologist, a podiatrist, a health educator, and others.

Fundamentals of Team Dynamics

Unfortunately, in today's work environment, team members' teamwork skills often lag far behind their technical skills. An understanding of the fundamentals of team dynamics, team development, team planning, team communication, and leadership sharing is an important adjunct to a professional's technical knowledge.

A team was previously defined in this chapter as "a small number of people with complementary skills who are committed to a common purpose, performance goals, and approach for which they hold themselves mutually accountable." Careful analysis of this definition reveals four important dimensions (**Figure 3–2**). First, a team should comprise a small number of people. Second, the team members must have complementary skills.

Third, there must be general consensus on why the team exists. Finally, the team members hold themselves mutually accountable for the work and results of the team's efforts.

Types of Teams

People are on groups and teams for many different reasons. Sometimes team membership is an end in itself. Many leisure activities lend themselves to team activities for the purpose of socializing. Cycling teams and basketball teams are just two examples of informal teams that satisfy social needs for working adults. Thus, an *informal team* can be defined as a team whose principal reason for existence is to provide friendship. People join such teams to have a sense of belonging, of acceptance, of recognition, and of being liked by others. Such teams usually do not have an officially appointed leader, although informal leadership often develops by popular acclaim. Informal teams usually develop spontaneously and may over time evolve into formal teams.[7]

Formal teams are created to achieve performance goals that, in turn, contribute to the success of the larger organization. Formal teams are more

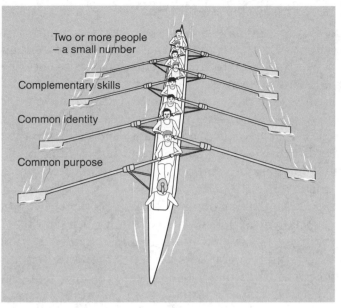

FIGURE 3–2 What does it take to make a team?

rationally structured and less fluid than informal ones. Rather than choosing to join, as in the case of informal teams, individuals are usually assigned to formal work teams because of their expertise and the needs of the team. One person is usually granted formal leadership responsibility.[7]

However, research has shown that in every high-performance team, leadership is shared.[5] This means that even though there is a designated leadership position, each member of the team shares responsibility for facilitating the team's work (**Figure 3–3**).

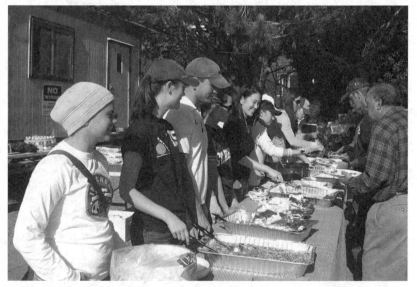

FIGURE 3–3 Nutrition students serving a lunch they prepared for a local labor exchange.
Courtesy of Lisa Ching, RD

Attraction to Teams, Roles, and Norms

Commitment to a team is said to hinge on two factors: attractiveness ("the outside looking in" view) and cohesiveness ("the inside looking out" view), or the tendency of the group to stick together and resist outside influences. A relatively small team of members who share similar traits with a high degree of interaction and cooperative relationships and who have a superior public image and enjoy prestige and status is the most likely to be attractive and cohesive. Unpleasant experiences and disagreements within the team, unreasonable demands made on team members, an unfavorable public image, and competition for membership and time all have a negative impact on attractiveness and cohesiveness.[8]

Also important to the functioning of a team is the concept of role. A **role** is defined as a socially determined prescription for behavior in a specific position. Every employee has one or more organizational roles to play. One key to organizational and team success is for everyone to play his or her role effectively and efficiently. Roles usually focus on a specific position, whereas norms are broader in scope.[9] **Norms** are general standards of conduct that help individuals judge what is right or wrong or good or bad; as such, they influence behavior enormously (**Figure 3–4**).[10]

Every team, whether informal or formal, develops its own set of norms that are enforced for the following reasons:

1. To ensure survival of the team
2. To simplify or clarify role expectations
3. To help team members avoid embarrassing situations and protect self-images
4. To express key team values and enhance the team's unique identification[11]

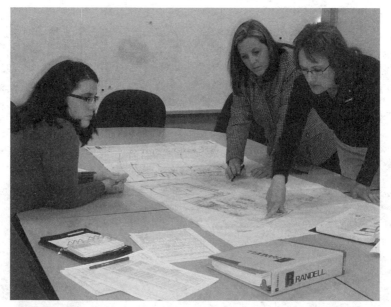

FIGURE 3–4 A facility design team, including a dietitian, collaborating on a project.
Courtesy of Christine Guyott, RD

Team Development

A group does not become a team overnight. The first few meetings of a new team may be fraught with a sense of uneasiness; lack of trust; uncertainty about roles, objectives, and leadership; and even defensive behavior and differences of opinion. Management experts have identified six stages of team development: orientation, conflict and challenge, cohesion, delusion, disillusion, and acceptance. During the first three stages, attempts are made to overcome uncertainty with regard to power and authority. Once this obstacle has been cleared, stages 4 through 6 address the uncertainty over interpersonal relationships. Teams that reach stage 6 are highly effective and efficient mature teams.[12]

The following are some important characteristics of mature teams:

1. Members are aware of their own and each other's assets and liabilities with regard to the team's task.
2. Individual differences are accepted without being labeled as good or bad.
3. The team has developed authority and interpersonal relationships that are recognized and accepted by the members.
4. Team decisions are made through rational discussion. Minority opinions and dissension are recognized and encouraged. Attempts are not made to force decisions or create a false unanimity.
5. Conflict is over substantive team issues such as team goals and the effectiveness and efficiency of various means for achieving those goals. Conflict over emotional issues regarding team structure, processes, or interpersonal relationships is at a minimum.
6. Members are aware of the team's processes and their own roles in them.[12]

Communicating for Team Success

Communication is the glue that binds the behavior among the members of the team. Communication can be defined as the constant development of understanding among people. Effective communication means that there is successful transfer of information, meaning, and understanding from a sender to a receiver. It is not necessary to have agreement, but there must be mutual understanding for the exchange to be considered successful.[13]

Types of Communication

Oral communication is the most common form of team communication and is generally superior to other forms of communication. Oral communication takes less time and is more effective in achieving understanding. Face-to-face communication has the advantage of also providing information through body language, personal mannerisms, and facial expressions.

Other types of communication include written communication, visual aids, gestures, and actions. Visual aids, such as pictures, charts, cartoons, symbols, and videos, can be particularly effective when used with good oral

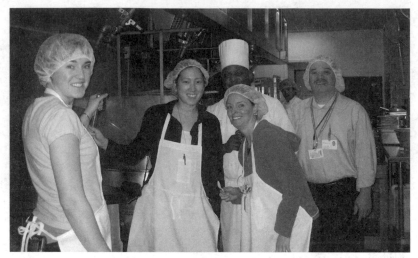

Figure 3–5 An executive chef, a foodservice manager, and interns team up on a meal project.
Courtesy of Jennifer Chang, RD

communication. "Actions speak louder than words" is sage advice for any manager. Gestures, handshakes, a shrug of the shoulders, a smile, and silence all have meaning and are powerful forms of communication to team members (**Figure 3–5**).

Barriers to Good Communication

Some barriers to communication have to do with the language used, the differing backgrounds of the sender and receiver, and the circumstances in which the communication takes place. The receiver may hear what he or she expects to hear and may shut out or ignore that which is unexpected or conflicts. The receiver also has a tendency to infer what is expected even when it is not communicated. Receivers are also susceptible to information overload, which occurs when someone receives more information than he or she is able to process.

Receivers evaluate the source and interpret or accept communication in light of that evaluation. A trusted and respected team member will have more open channels of communication than a team member who does not command trust and respect.

Different people often attach various meanings to certain words. The sender or communicator not only must choose words that convey the meaning to the receiver, but also must give attention to the message transmitted by nonverbal cues. Body language and facial expression often say more than the words they accompany.

A receiver who is emotionally upset often stops listening in order to think about what he or she will say next. Noise and the environment may form a physical barrier to communication. Time and place are also important. There is a right place and a wrong place to conduct good communication, just as there is a right time and a wrong time. Time pressures on the sender form a barrier to effective communication because of hastily developed messages, use of the most expedient rather than the most effective channel, and insufficient time for feedback.

A network breakdown occurs when there is a disruption or closure of a communication channel. This can be caused by a number of factors, both intentional and unintentional. Some factors that can cause the network to break down are forgetfulness, jealousy, fear of negative feedback, and a desire to gain an edge over the competition.

Improving Communication

Communication is not a one-way process. One of the most important parts of effective communication is to listen to the reply, which may entail words, facial expressions, body language, and even silence. The evaluation of feedback can tell much about how the message has been received. Empathy—the ability to put yourself in the receiver's shoes in a conversation—is crucial to mutual understanding.

Face-to-face communication is advantageous because of the ability to gain immediate feedback from multiple channels, such as oral expression, facial expressions, and body language. To secure understanding, it is often effective to repeat the information using slightly different words, phrases, or approaches. Being sensitive to the receiver can improve communication. Some words or phrases have symbolic meaning to others, and these words should be avoided. Proper timing is also important. The old maxim "criticize in private, praise in public" is an example of timing. Reinforcing words with congruent actions has already been discussed as essential to effective communication. Finally, an atmosphere of openness and trust, fostered by self-disclosure, builds healthy relationships that contribute to effective communication in a team setting.[13]

Productive Communication

Teamwork requires productive communication that supports and encourages authentic, inclusive sharing and negotiation of ideas and perspectives. When this occurs, a climate develops in which members are sensitive to one another, dialogue is supported, and defensiveness is reduced through language that is **assertive, responsible, confirming,** and **appropriate.**[13]

Sensitivity means being able to understand other team members' feelings and responses and to adapt the response accordingly. People who are able to do this are flexible, assertive, and not bound by predetermined gender roles.[14]

Note that assertiveness is not aggressiveness. Aggressive communication is an attempt to control others, with a low regard for their interests or feelings. **Assertive communication** is open, with an awareness of self and concern for others. Even though assertiveness is often direct, it is also very gentle and considerate of others' opinions. Team members who are assertive focus on problems, not on people, and on openness, not on strategy or manipulation. Being assertive means taking some risks, knowing and stating your position responsibly and openly, and being sensitive to others' responses.

Responsible communication means taking responsibility for one's feelings and ideas. Some years ago, it was suggested that "I statements" are a more responsible way of communicating. Starting a statement with "you" rather than "I" implies that someone else is to blame; for example, saying "You're always late" versus "I feel frustrated that you are often late." Absolute terms such as "always" and "never" should also be avoided.[15]

Confirming communication means listening to, acknowledging, and understanding the ideas and feelings of others. This is often accomplished with statements like "That's a good idea" or "Tell us more about that." Such statements are called person-centered messages, and they confirm a person's worth and role in a process. A person who uses person-centered messages is seen as more persuasive.[16] The opposite of confirmation is rejection or disconfirming, which may be communicated with silence, changing the subject, or an impersonal response.[17]

Appropriate communication means using dialogue that opens up the discussion and understanding. It means using language that fits the team members, yourself, and the team context. Appropriate communication means being clear and concrete and speaking at the listeners' knowledge level.[3]

A team that has mastered the art of productive communication should be able to say:

- We support and confirm one another so that everyone speaks and is heard.
- We respect one another's differences and adapt our communication to open up discussion.
- We take care to express our ideas responsibly and appropriately.
- We consider and refine our thinking with careful negotiation and definition of terms.[3]

What Makes a Work Team Effective?

Based on a number of studies, the determinants of team effectiveness may be grouped into three categories: people-related factors, organization-related factors, and task-related factors.

People-Related Factors
> Personal work satisfaction
> Mutual trust and team spirit
> Good communication
> Low unresolved conflict and power struggle
> Low threat, fail-safe, good job security

Organization-Related Factors
> Organizational stability and job security
> Involved, interested, supportive management
> Stable goals and priorities

Task-Related Factors
> Clear objectives, directions, and plans
> Proper technical direction and leadership

Autonomy and professionally challenging work
Experienced and qualified team personnel
Team involvement and work visibility

The presence of these determinants leads to effective team performance characterized by:

- Accomplishment of goals
- Adaptability to change
- High personal/team commitment
- High rating by upper management
- Generation of innovative ideas[18]

Among the people-related factors, one stands out as being key to effective teamwork and requires careful attention in today's work milieu—trust. **Trust** is the belief in the integrity, character, or ability of others. Trust is a fragile entity. Earning a person's trust is a long, slow process that can be destroyed in an instant with a careless remark. In the team process, the primary responsibility for building a climate of trust belongs to the team leader, but each member of the team shares this responsibility. There are six ways to build trust:

- **Communication.** Be open and honest, provide timely feedback, and keep people informed.
- **Support.** Be approachable and available to help, encourage, and coach.
- **Respect.** Delegate important duties and be a good listener.
- **Fairness.** Evaluate people fairly and objectively; be liberal in giving credit and praise.
- **Predictability.** Be dependable and consistent in your behavior; keep promises and deadlines.
- **Competence.** Be technically and professionally competent; be a good role model.

Although concentration on these six areas is advised for team leaders, they are equally important for team members. In addition, those who feel trusted tend to trust others in return.[7]

Members of Healthcare Teams

There are more than 100 possible members of the healthcare team![19] This section highlights a few of the professionals who may be included on the healthcare team. Members of the dietetic team form a subset of the larger healthcare team and are discussed first. Members of the dietetic team can most often be found working in the organizational healthcare setting. Dietitians, dietetic technicians, and dietary managers are the primary positions that make up the dietetic team. In recent years, healthcare issues such as labor shortages, cost containment, and quality assurance have forced the dietetic team to be better coordinated and to delegate less specialized, more routine tasks to less highly trained personnel.

Dietitians

Dietitians are highly qualified professionals who are recognized experts on food and nutrition. The educational requirements to become a dietitian are described in Chapter 5. The Academy of Nutrition and Dietetics is the primary professional association for dietitians and dietetic technicians. Dietitians work in a wide variety of settings, most of which fall into nine categories, discussed next.

Dietitians in Business.   Dietitians in business work in areas such as food manufacturing, advertising, and marketing. Dietitians who work for food manufacturers or grocery chains may analyze the nutrition content for foods for labeling purposes or marketing efforts. They may also prepare literature for distribution to customers and write articles for the news media. To satisfy consumers' growing interest in nutrition, dietitians are employed by businesses to develop new products, sell and market products, and develop public relations and advertising programs. Many entrepreneurial dietitians have developed a product, product line, or service themselves and have built a company to market and sell the products or services (**Figure 3–6**).

Clinical Dietitians.   Clinical dietitians provide nutritional services for patients in hospitals, nursing homes, clinics, health maintenance organizations (HMOs), doctors' offices, and other healthcare facilities. They assess patients' nutritional needs, develop and implement nutrition programs, and evaluate and report the results. They are a vital part of the healthcare team, working with doctors and other healthcare professionals to coordinate nutritional intake with other treatments, such as medications (**Figure 3–7**).

Many clinical dietitians specialize in one area of practice. Diabetes, heart disease, pediatrics, geriatrics, renal disease, the critically ill, and obesity are some of the areas in which clinical dietitians specialize. Nutritional care of the critically ill, for example, involves overseeing patients requiring tube or intravenous feedings. Clinical dietitians working with patients with diabetes

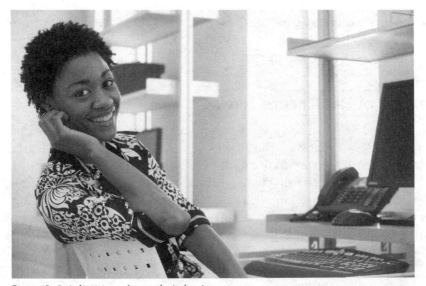

FIGURE 3–6 A dietitian who works in business.
© bikeriderlondon/Shutterstock

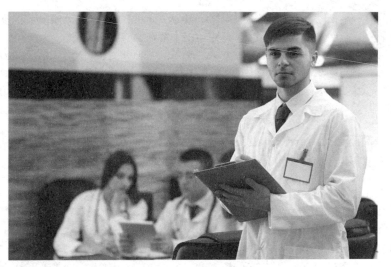

FIGURE 3–7 A clinical dietitian.
© Africa Studio/Shutterstock

teach them how to establish and adhere to a long-term nutrition program and how to monitor blood glucose levels.

In addition to assessing patients' nutrition needs and developing treatment plans, clinical dietitians have administrative and managerial duties. In a small nursing home or hospital, the clinical dietitian may run the foodservice department. In larger facilities, the clinical dietitian may supervise dietetic technicians and other support staff such as patient service supervisors, diet clerks, and clerical personnel.

Community Dietitians.   Community dietitians reach out to the public to teach, monitor, and advise individuals and groups in their efforts to prevent

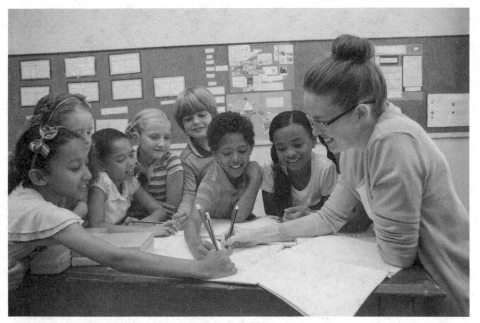

FIGURE 3–8 A community dietitian working with children.
© wavebreakmedia/Shutterstock

disease and promote good health (**Figure 3–8**). They are employed by international organizations; federal, state, and local governments; food businesses; and trade associations. A variety of public, private, and volunteer organizations concerned with international health employ community nutritionists. The United Nations and the Peace Corps are just two such organizations. The U.S. Department of Agriculture, the U.S. Department of Health and Human Services, and the public health division of state and local governments employ community nutritionists to plan and carry out programs to address nutritional problems of targeted groups. The WIC (Women, Infants, and Children) program is one example. The main responsibility of community nutritionists employed by food businesses and associations is nutrition education. For example, the dairy industry has organized large-scale nutrition education programs for schoolchildren and other groups.

Community dietitians evaluate individual needs, establish nutritional care plans, and communicate the principles of good nutrition in a way that individuals and their families can understand. Teaching is a very large component of the community dietitian's job. Topics run the gamut, ranging from grocery shopping to the preparation of infant formula. They also support menu planning for those with diabetes, alcoholism, or hypertension, among many other conditions.

Consultant Dietitians.   Consultant dietitians may be self-employed in their own private practice or under contract to one or more healthcare facilities. In private practice, the consultant dietitian performs nutrition screening and assessment of clients, who are often referred by a physician. Weight loss is the most common diet-related concern of clients who seek a private-practice dietitian. Consultant dietitians under contract to healthcare facilities

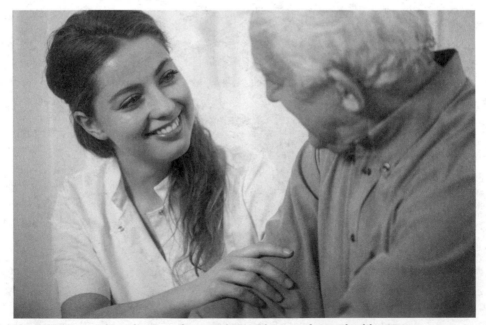

FIGURE 3–9 A consultant dietitian who specializes in the area of senior health.
© Photographee.eu/Shutterstock

provide expert advice on foodservice management issues such as menu planning, budgeting, cost control, portion control, sanitation, and safety. They also monitor clinical nutritional care (**Figure 3–9**).

Dietitians in Education.   Dietitians in education teach the science of food and nutrition to future dietitians, dietetic technicians, dietary managers, doctors, nurses, dentists, chefs, and others. Their employers are universities, colleges, community colleges, technical schools, medical schools, dietetic internship programs, and other educational programs. Although education is a major component of most dietitians' job responsibilities, this category is for those who are employed by an educational institution or program, rather than an organization whose primary responsibility is health care.

Management Dietitians.   Although management is a major component of most dietitians' job responsibilities, this category is for those who have the title of manager, director, or administrator. They are responsible for large-scale meal planning and preparation in such places as hospitals, nursing homes, retirement residences, company cafeterias, correctional facilities, elementary and secondary schools, food factories, colleges and universities, transportation companies, restaurants, the military, and recreational facilities.

The management dietitian supervises the planning, preparation, and service of meals; selects, trains, and directs other dietitians, foodservice supervisors, and foodservice workers; budgets for and purchases food, equipment, and supplies; enforces sanitary and safety regulations; prepares records and reports; and directs clinical services, public health nutrition, and other nutrition programs.

Dietitians who direct food and nutrition departments also decide on departmental policies and coordinate food and nutrition services with the activities of other departments. The use of computer programs to adjust recipes, prepare purchase orders, cost recipes and menus, keep inventory records, prepare financial reports, conduct nutritional analyses, and so on, has simplified many of the routine functions of management dietetics.

Research Dietitians.   Research dietitians work for government agencies, food or pharmaceutical companies, academic medical centers, or educational institutions. Using the scientific method and analytical techniques, they conduct studies that range from pure to applied science. Often the research is conducted collaboratively with physicians, exercise physiologists, chemists, food technologists, and researchers from other disciplines. Research dietitians may explore the way the body uses a particular food or the interaction of drugs and diet. They may investigate the nutritional needs of individuals with different diseases or ways to reduce the risk of disease. Research in the management arena may involve the effectiveness of various foodservice systems or the efficiency of different types of foodservice equipment.

Dietetic Technicians.   Dietetic technicians complete a 2-year associate degree in an Academy of Nutrition and Dietetics–approved dietetic technician program that combines both classroom and supervised practice experiences. They are then eligible to take the registration examination for dietetic technicians. Individuals who pass the exam may then use the initials NDTR, for Nutrition and Dietetics Technician, Registered, after their name.

Dietetic technicians work in a wide variety of settings and assume an even wider variety of responsibilities. Dietetic technicians are found in hospitals, public health nutrition programs, long-term care facilities, child nutrition and school lunch programs, nutrition programs for the elderly, and foodservice management. Screening patients to identify nutritional problems, modifying menus, providing patient education and counseling to individuals and groups, developing menus and recipes, supervising foodservice personnel, purchasing food, conducting inventory, and maintaining computer systems are the most commonly performed functions of a dietetic technician.

Dietary Managers.   Dietary managers are members of the Association of Nutrition & Foodservice Professionals (ANFP), formerly the Dietary Managers Association (DMA). Although no legal relationship exists between the Academy of Nutrition and Dietetics and the ANFP, a very close working relationship has always existed. Dietary managers have been trained in foodservice operations and usually supervise and manage dietetic service in long-term care facilities, hospitals, schools, the military, correctional institutions, and other noncommercial foodservice operations.

Other Members of the Healthcare Team

A few of the more than 100 members of the healthcare team are highlighted in this section.

Physicians.   Required training for physicians includes a 4-year postgraduate medical degree (either an MD or a DO). Medical schools in the United States have specific undergraduate entrance requirements, including coursework in mathematics, the sciences, and the humanities. Entrance to medical school is very competitive and is based on undergraduate gradepoint average, the results of a standardized medical school entrance exam, letters of recommendation, and community service, volunteer, or research experience.

Medical school includes 2 years of basic medical science followed by 2 years of clinical training. The clinical training concentrates heavily on the daily care of hospitalized patients. During these 2 years, medical students begin to explore areas of specialization in medicine. After graduation from medical school, doctors are required to complete a residency in a specialty, which lasts 3 to 5 years. A fellowship may follow the residency program if a doctor wants to train in a subspecialty area. For example, a residency in pediatrics could be followed by a fellowship in neonatology (care of newborns, including premature infants), pediatric cardiology (the heart and circulatory system), pediatric neurology (the brain and nervous system), pediatric hematology (the blood), pediatric oncology (cancer and tumors), pediatric gastroenterology (the digestive system), or pediatric nephrology (the kidneys).

- **Cardiology.** Cardiologists diagnose and treat cardiovascular defects and diseases. They are concerned with the structure and function of the heart and blood vessels and with the circulation of blood throughout the body.
- **Emergency medicine.** An emergency physician focuses on the immediate decision making and action necessary to prevent death or any

further disability in the emergency room. The emergency physician provides immediate recognition, evaluation, care, stabilization, and disposition of patients in response to acute illness and injury.

- **Endocrinology.** An endocrinologist diagnoses and treats diseases of the hormone-producing glandular system—including the pituitary, thyroid, parathyroid, and adrenal glands and the gonads—and the insulin-producing cells of the pancreas. Endocrinologists also treat patients with metabolic disorders.

- **Family practice.** A family physician is concerned with the total health of the individual and the family and is trained to diagnose and treat a wide variety of ailments in patients of all ages. The family physician's broad training includes internal medicine, pediatrics, obstetrics and gynecology, psychiatry, and geriatrics. Special emphasis is placed on prevention and the primary care of entire families.

- **Internal medicine.** An internist provides long-term comprehensive care in the office and the hospital, managing both common and complex illnesses of all ages. Internists are trained in diagnosis and treatment of cancer, infections, and diseases affecting the heart, blood, kidneys, joints, and digestive, respiratory, and vascular systems. They are also trained in the essentials of primary care internal medicine, which includes an understanding of disease prevention, wellness, substance abuse, mental health, and the effective treatment of common problems of the eyes, ears, skin, nervous system, and reproductive organs.

- **Neurology.** An internal medicine specialty, neurology deals with disorders of the human brain, spinal cord, peripheral nerves, and muscles. Neurologists care for patients with a myriad of disorders such as pain, weakness in the arms or legs, or memory loss.

- **Obstetrics/gynecology.** An obstetrician/gynecologist has special knowledge, skills, and professional capability in the medical and surgical care of the female reproductive system and associated disorders.

- **Oncology.** An oncologist is concerned with neoplastic growth (abnormal new growth of cells and tissues), including the cause and the pattern of the abnormality.

- **Ophthalmology.** An ophthalmologist deals with the structure, function, and diseases of the eye, including medical and surgical treatment of its defects and diseases.

- **Osteopathy.** Osteopathy is a system of medical practice based on a theory that diseases are due chiefly to loss of structural integrity that can be restored by manipulation of the affected parts, supplemented by therapeutic measures (e.g., medicine, physical therapy, or surgery). During medical school, osteopathic physicians (DOs) receive extra training in the musculoskeletal system (the body's interconnected system of nerves, muscles, and bones that make up about two-thirds of the body mass). DOs are trained to be primary care physicians with a focus on preventive health care. They practice a "whole-person" approach to medicine; rather than treating specific symptoms or illnesses, they assess the overall health of the person, including home and work environments.

- **Pathology.** Pathologists provide and interpret laboratory information to help solve diagnostic problems and monitor the effects of therapy for other medical specialists.
- **Pediatrics.** Pediatricians provide preventive health maintenance for healthy children and medical care for those who are ill. Pediatricians diagnose and treat infections, injuries, genetic defects, malignancies, and many types of organic disease and dysfunction.
- **Psychiatry.** Psychiatrists specialize in the prevention, diagnosis, and treatment of mental, addictive, and emotional disorders such as schizophrenia and other psychotic, mood, anxiety, substance-related, sexual and gender identity, and adjustment disorders.
- **Surgery.** Surgeons deal with problems by using operative procedures. The problems may be mechanical or structural (e.g., hernias, fractures, ulcers), biological (e.g., ulcers), or metabolic (e.g., an islet cell tumor of the pancreas, which causes the pancreas to secrete too much insulin). Surgical subspecialties include gastrointestinal (digestive tract), plastic surgery, vascular (blood vessels), cardiothoracic (heart and chest), pediatric (infants and children), endocrine (glands), orthopedic (bones and nervous system), otolaryngology (ear, nose, and throat), gynecology (female organs), hand, trauma and burn, oncology (cancer), and transplantation (transplanted organs).

Nurses. Registered nurses (RNs) are active in the prevention of illness in clinics, industry, and public health; the care of patients in emergency and intensive-care settings; and the care of patients in their own homes. There are more than 100 nursing specialties. The specialty may focus on a specific disease, organ/system, work setting, scope of practice, patient age, criticalness of patient condition, or technology.

NURSE PRACTITIONERS. Nurse practitioners are registered nurses with advanced formal education. Most have a master's degree in nursing and are certified by a national professional association. Working in collaboration with physicians and other members of the healthcare team, nurse practitioners obtain medical histories and perform physical exams; diagnose and treat common health problems; diagnose, treat, and monitor chronic diseases; order and interpret lab work and x-rays; provide family planning, prenatal care, well-baby and child care, and health maintenance care; conduct patient and family education and counseling programs; provide referrals to healthcare team members; and, in some states, prescribe medication.

LICENSED PRACTICAL/VOCATIONAL NURSES. Licensed practical nurses (LPNs), or licensed vocational nurses (LVNs), as they are called in California and Texas, provide basic bedside care by taking vital signs, treating bedsores, preparing and giving injections and enemas, monitoring catheters, observing patients, collecting samples for testing, feeding patients, and recording food and fluid intake and output. They also help patients with bathing, dressing, and personal hygiene.

CERTIFIED NURSING ASSISTANTS. Certified nursing assistants (CNAs) perform various patient/resident care activities and related nursing functions necessary to provide for the personal needs and comfort of the facility residents/

patients. CNA duties include serving meals, nourishments, and liquids; assisting in feeding those in need of help; taking vital signs and reporting abnormal findings; and participating actively in all routine hygiene procedures related to resident care.

Physician Assistants. The physician assistant (PA), under the supervision of a physician, performs diagnostic, therapeutic, preventive, and health maintenance services. Working as members of the healthcare team, PAs take medical histories, examine patients, order and interpret laboratory reports and x-rays, and make diagnoses. They also treat minor injuries by suturing, splinting, and casting. PAs record progress notes, instruct and counsel patients, and order or carry out therapy. In almost every state, PAs may prescribe medications.

Pharmacists. Hospital pharmacists monitor a patient's drug therapy, prepare intravenous medications and feedings, oversee drug administration, and make purchasing decisions. Pharmacists are important members of many healthcare teams.

Social Workers. The field of social work is incredibly broad. A bachelor of arts in social work is always required; a master's degree in social work (MSW) is increasingly required. The undergraduate degree is broad-based, with elective courses in substance abuse, grief, and race and gender issues. Graduate programs explore human behavior, mental disorders, and methods of intervention and psychotherapy in greater depth.

Chiropractors. A doctor of chiropractic (DC) has completed a minimum of 2 years of college credit toward a baccalaureate degree and 3 to 4 years at a chiropractic college. Chiropractic emphasizes a holistic approach to health and is based on the premise that the relationship between structure and function in the human body (particularly of the spinal column and nervous system) is a significant health factor. Chiropractors believe that when the spinal column is out of alignment the body's natural defenses against disease and illness are lowered. Chiropractors realign the spinal column so that the body stays in a state of homeostasis, or balance.

Physical Therapists. Physical therapists design and administer rehabilitative exercise programs for people with injuries or disabilities that affect their daily functioning.

Athletic Trainers. Athletic trainers provide services such as injury prevention, recognition, immediate care, treatment, and rehabilitation of athletic trauma.

Occupational Therapists. Occupational therapists and their assistants provide service to individuals whose abilities to cope with the tasks of living are threatened or impaired by developmental deficits, the aging process, poverty and cultural differences, physical injury or illness, or psychological and social disability. The therapy is directed toward teaching adaptive skills and enhancing performance capacity to achieve optimal function, prevent disability, or maintain health. The goal is the highest possible functional independence for self-care, work, and leisure.

Speech-Language Pathologists. Speech-language pathologists assess, diagnose, treat, and help prevent speech, language, cognitive, communication, voice, swallowing, and fluency problems. Specifically related to dietetics, speech-language pathologists work with people who have oral motor problems that cause eating and swallowing difficulties.

Medical Laboratory Technicians/Technologists. Under the supervision of a pathologist, a "lab tech" performs lab tests, using precision instruments, on blood, tissues, and body fluids to detect, diagnose, and treat diseases. Medical lab technologists are able to perform the same duties as a technician and can also perform more complex analyses, discrimination, and detection of errors. Histologic technicians/technologists specialize in the preparation of body tissues for laboratory analysis.

Radiologic Technologists. Under the supervision of radiation oncologists, "rad techs" administer radiation therapy to patients. Radiographers, also under the supervision of qualified physicians, provide patient service using imaging modalities.

Nuclear Medicine Technologists. A nuclear medicine technologist assists a nuclear medicine physician. These physicians use the nuclear properties of radioactive and stable nuclides to make diagnostic evaluations of the anatomic or physiologic conditions of the body.

Respiratory Therapists. The respiratory therapist and respiratory therapy technician evaluate all data to determine the appropriate respiratory care for a patient and conduct the therapeutic procedures to carry out this plan.

Medical Assistants

Medical assistants assist physicians in their offices or other medical settings by performing a variety of administrative and clinical duties.

Medical Records Administrators. A medical record comprises the complete and permanent documents maintained for every person treated in a medical facility. Medical records administrators manage the medical record in compliance with medical, administrative, ethical, and legal requirements. The medical records technician (MRT) is responsible for maintaining the medical records.

Summary

Management guru Ken Blanchard wisely observed, "None of us is as smart as all of us." Teamwork is important in the healthcare professions today, partly because of the enormous number of people employed in these careers. The team approach is an effective way of dealing with the fragmentation of care that may occur because of specialization.

Teamwork may be problematic if roles are not clearly defined, communication is not adequate and open, members fail to be good team players, and team goals are not clearly defined. Accurate and timely sharing of data is a key element in the effectiveness of the team effort. Team conferences, in which all team members share information and participate in decision making, are the preferred approach.

Dietitians, dietetic technicians, and dietary managers are the members of the dietetic team. They have all received formal training in foods and nutrition, and, as a team, they work in a wide variety of settings. Dietitians, who are recognized experts in food and nutrition, are found working in the business, clinical, community, consulting, education, management, and research arenas. Dietetic technicians must complete a 2-year associate degree in an Academy of Nutrition and Dietetics–approved dietetic technician program and then pass the registration examination for dietetic technicians. Dietary managers complete a 1-year college course.

Effective teamwork requires shared goals, clearly defined roles, and a plan for coordinating efforts. Whenever possible, the patient should be part of the team. Any health professional can testify to the importance of patient cooperation in the diagnostic, therapeutic, and rehabilitative processes.

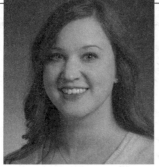

Courtesy of Karen Brtko

Profile of a Professional

Karen Brtko, DTR

Clinical Dietetic Technician
Cincinnati Children's Hospital Medical Center, Cincinnati, Ohio

Education:
Cincinnati State Technical and Community College, Cincinnati, Ohio

How did you first hear about dietetics and decide to become a Dietetic Technician, Registered?
I've always wanted to work in healthcare but wasn't sure where I fit in. At one time, I had been working with children in a gymnastics program. Seeing firsthand the nutritional challenges that children face today, I researched a career in dietetics and found my niche.

What was your route to registration?
I went the traditional route and completed a 2-year dietetics technician program that included supervised practice experiences.

In what types of facilities did you gain your supervised practice experience?
As a student, I gained experience in many different settings including acute care, long-term care, pediatrics, and also food service management and culinary. For me, the best part about my education was the hands-on learning aspect. With the supervised practice requirements, you're not only learning about subjects, but also learning how to apply your knowledge in a professional setting.

How have you been involved professionally?
I've been fortunate to have been invited to volunteer with the Academy, Commission on Dietetic Registration (CDR), and Accreditation Council for Education in Nutrition and Dietetics (ACEND) on different occasions. I participated in item writing for the DTR registration exam. I also sat on a focus group about changes in the Professional Development Portfolio. Most recently I was invited to be on a task force for the 2015 Dietetics Practice Audit. The opportunity to collaborate with other dietetics professionals on the national level is an experience I'd highly recommend to anyone in the field.

Briefly describe your career path in dietetics. What are you doing now?
I have a wonderful job at Cincinnati Children's Hospital Medical Center. As a clinical diet tech, I provide direct patient care and I support registered dietitians (RDs) in the acute care inpatient setting. The best part about my job is that it's different every day. There is always an opportunity to learn something new, get involved, and improve patient outcomes.

What excites you about dietetics and the future of our profession?
Dietetics is an exciting profession because nutrition plays a role in everyone's life. I think people view good nutrition as more of a priority today than in the past because healthy eating is now widely viewed as a measure of preventative care. I think that

as science progresses, nutrition experts are becoming more of a key presence within the medical team, the corporate world, and the general public. And the list keeps growing.

How is teamwork important to you in your position? How have you been involved in team projects?

The presence of a nutrition team in healthcare gives the patient and his/her family a sense of security with regard to a treatment plan. RDs and DTRs have unique roles that are built to support each other and to implement the nutrition plan for the patient. Teamwork and communication are essential to providing the best possible outcomes for treatment. Teamwork extends beyond patient care as well. As a DTR, I have been involved in councils and committees, gathered data for research studies, mentored students, and participated in multidisciplinary meetings.

What words of wisdom do you have for future dietetics professionals?

Be a leader. As a nutrition expert, your knowledge is valuable. Don't be afraid to offer your expertise and insight where it may be needed.

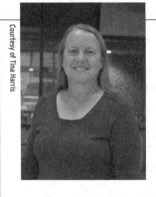

Courtesy of Tina Harris

Profile of a Professional

Tina Harris, MA, RD, LD

Clinical Nutrition Manager

Morrison Healthcare at NEA Baptist Hospital, Jonesboro, Arkansas

Education:

BS in Dietetics, Black River Technical College, Pocahontas, Arkansas, and the University of Medicine and Dentistry of New Jersey, Newark, New Jersey MA in Organizational Management, Ashford University, Clinton, Iowa

How did you first hear about dietetics and decide to become a Registered Dietitian?

This was a very gradual process for me, but I will try and keep it brief. I worked at a shoe factory for 15 years and then the factory was moved to Mexico. I was given the choice to draw unemployment and go to college for 2 years or just find another job. Our local college, Black River Technical College, has a dietetic program that offers dietary manager and dietetic technician programs. I loved to cook, so I decided to go to college and see where it would take me. I started taking classes and became a certified dietary manager (CDM) and continued to take classes to finish my 2-year degree. I was running out of unemployment, so I opened a restaurant so I could finish my last semester of college. I hired other dietetic students who had different class schedules to work for me during my class hours. I eventually sold the restaurant and worked as a DTR for long-term care (LTC) for 2 years. In 2000, Black River Technical College offered me a job managing their cafeteria and teaching classes for the dietary managers program.

What was your route to registration?

I chose to finish my dietetics degree online at the University of Medicine and Dentistry of New Jersey (UMDNJ; now Rutgers University), a coordinated program.

At what college did your receive your entry-level education?

Black River Technical College for my CDM and DTR credentials and UMDNJ for my RD credential.

Where did you complete your supervised practice?

I had contracts with Health South Rehab, St. Bernard's Medical Center, and NEA Baptist Hospital, which are all located in Jonesboro, Arkansas. I completed my community rotations at Brad Head Start and NEA Food Bank, which are located in Pocahontas, Arkansas.

Do you have an advanced degree?

I have a Master of Arts in Organizational Management with emphasis in Leadership from Ashford University in Clinton, Iowa.

What are some examples of your professional involvement at the local, state, or national level in dietetic-related professional associations?

- District President of Dietary Managers Association, 2003–2004
- State Treasurer of Dietary Managers Association, 2007
- State Secretary of Dietary Managers Association, 2008
- Dietary Managers Association, State Legislative Committee, Washington, DC trip, 2008
- Website Coordinator for Arkansas Dietary Managers Association, 2009
- District President of Arkansas Dietetics Association, 2009–2010
- President-Elect of Dietary Managers Association, 2009
- Arkansas Dietary Managers Association State President, 2010
- State Treasurer for Association of Nutrition & Foodservice Professionals (ANFP), 2012–2016
- Program Reviewer for ANFP, 2010–2013
- ANFP Item Writer Committee for CDM, Certified Food Protection Professional (CFPP) exam, 2011–2012
- Program Chair for ANFP, 2011–2013
- Preceptor for University of Medicine and Dentistry of New Jersey students, 2009–present in food security, diabetes and community, rotations
- Preceptor for Arkansas State University dietetics students present

What honors and awards have you received?

- Phi Theta Kappa Society, GPA 3.95
- Arkansas Dietetic Technician of the Year 1999–2000
- Black River Technical College Faculty of the Year 2003
- Platinum Dietary Manager's State Achievement Award 2010
- Recognized for continued commitment to leadership by Association of Nutrition & Foodservice Professionals 2015

Briefly describe your career path in dietetics. What are you doing now?

I began teaching for Black River Technical College (BRTC) in 2000 and started taking classes toward my bachelor's degree in 2005. Once I graduated and passed the RD exam, I started consulting part-time for two local nursing homes and NEA Baptist, where I am now employed. I was also promoted to Program Director for Dietetics at BRTC.

I decided to become more diverse with my education and started taking classes toward my master's degree in 2009. Once I finished my master's degree, I was promoted to the Business Department Head as well as keeping my other responsibilities at BRTC.

As I mentioned before, I had started working part-time for NEA Baptist Hospital in 2007. In 2012, they offered me a position as Clinical Nutrition Manager in a new facility, and I accepted. I enjoy my job because I do feel like I make a difference in someone's life daily. I also continue to precept for Arkansas State University, Rutgers (formerly UMDNJ), and BRTC students, which lets me fulfill my need to teach.

What excites you about dietetics and the future of our profession?

It could be just because I am interested in dietetics but I have noticed that people seem more interested in how nutrition plays a part in maintaining good health. In the past few years, nutrition has even been promoted by our First Lady, Michelle Obama, and been a controversial issue in school lunch programs. I am excited when nutrition is brought up in any situation because it can then become a teachable moment. I truly believe that our profession will continue to gain respect in the medical field and more people will have a better understanding of what dietetics really involves.

How is teamwork important to you in your position? How have you been involved in team projects?

My position revolves around teamwork; our management team requires each member to be responsible and reliable to make the department run as one. We all have different ways of working out problems, but at the end of the day, we are all responsible for each other's results.

I always try to stay involved with community projects and support groups outside of work. This experience allows me to relate to others on a different level. I like to work with volunteer groups where we can work together to help others without the pressure of being perfect or graded on how we perform. I volunteer to present/speak at district, state, and local meetings, cancer support groups, Head Start programs, and libraries, and have done cooking demos for rural communities.

What words of wisdom do you have for future dietetics professional?

I was given this advice once and I try to pass it on: Always know your strengths and weaknesses, and then build your team to complement them. You can then learn from each other and be a strong team.

Suggested Activities

1. Find out what's new with teams and teamwork. Teams are becoming an increasingly more important part of organizational life, and, as a result, much is changing in this area. Go to the Tips 4 Teamwork website at www.tips4teamwork.com. Click the "Articles" main menu tab on the homepage. Select and read at least two of the full-text articles and find at least three good ideas for successful teamwork. Share these with your classmates.

2. How good of a team player are you? Could you become a better team player? Which of your teamwork skills need improvement? Think of a team you are currently on or a team you may have been on in the past and take the quiz at www.mindtools.com. Were you surprised by the results? How will this self-knowledge be of help to you in forming or working on a team?

3. Want to improve your teamwork or communication skills? Go to www.gamesforgroups.com; under the Therapeutic Games tab, click the "Teamwork Activities" or the "Communication Activities" links. Gather the materials needed. With a group of classmates, try some of the teamwork and communication exercises.

4. Contact a large medical center or hospital in your area to see whether it has a dietetic team. Talk to the members of the team to determine their roles and responsibilities in delivering nutritional care to clients.

5. With a team of fellow students, write a paper on the principles of teamwork. In doing the research and writing the paper, apply the principles that have been found to be effective. Evaluate your success as a team. What worked well and why? What didn't work and why?

6. Choose any of the allied health professions. Do an in-depth study of its educational requirements, job responsibilities, areas of specialization, and so on.

7. Visit a local hospital cafeteria, and talk to as many of its employees as you can. Try to determine if, how, and to what extent they work with members of the dietetic team.

8. Volunteer to work in a hospital or other healthcare facility. This is an excellent way to learn about various healthcare professions and to help those who need it at the same time.

9. Are you interested in the salaries offered for the different allied health professions? The Bureau of Labor Statistics gathers employment and wage data periodically and reports it on its website. Go to www.bls .gov and compare the wage estimates shown. Which states and metropolitan areas offer the highest salaries?

10. Are you a good communicator? Communication is such an everyday activity that it is seldom given much thought. This activity is an opportunity to assess your communication style and skills to see how you might become a more effective communicator. Visit the website www .queendom.com. Click the main menu category "Tests." Under "Relationship Tests," click "Interpersonal Communication Skills Test." Were you surprised by the results? What are your strengths and limitations, and what do you need to do to improve?

Selected Websites

- www.aapa.org—American Academy of Physician Assistants
- www.ama-assn.org—American Medical Association
- www.bls.gov—U.S. Bureau of Labor Statistics
- www.fastcompany.com—Site features full-text magazine articles on teamwork and team building
- www.gamesforgroups.com—Site features therapeutic and team-building games
- www.mindtools.com—Site features a quiz to assess team effectiveness
- www.osteopathic.org—American Osteopathic Association
- www.queendom.com—Site offers a variety of online tests
- www.teambuildersplus.com—Team Builders Plus helps individuals develop the skills to create a team environment.

Suggested Readings

Damp DV. *Health Care Job Explosion! High Growth Health Care Careers and Job Locator*, 3rd ed. Moon Township, PA: Bookhaven Press LLC; 2001.

Fazio Maruca R. What makes teams work. Fast Company. October 31, 2000. Available at: http://www.fastcompany.com/41112/what-makes-teams-work. Accessed March 18, 2016.

Fishman C. The Whole Foods recipe for teamwork. Fast Company. April 31, 1996. Available at: http://www.fastcompany.com/26641/whole-foods-recipe-teamwork. Accessed March18, 2016.

Kouzes JM, Posner BZ. *The Leadership Challenge*, 4th ed. San Francisco: Jossey-Bass; 2007.

Levi D. *Group Dynamics for Teams*. Thousand Oaks, CA: Sage; 2001.

Moores S. Six heads are better than one. *ADA Times* 2003;1(1):1–3.

Roberts P. The agenda—total teamwork. Fast Company. March 31, 1999. Available at: http://www.fastcompany.com/36969/agenda-total-teamwork. Accessed March18, 2016.

Stanfield P, Hui YH. *Introduction to the Health Professions*. Burlington, MA: Jones and Bartlett Learning; 2012.

References

1. Reprinted from *Journal of the American Dietetic Association*, 96, Number 12 (December 1996), George I. Balch, "Employers' Perceptions of the Roles of Dietetics Practitioners: Challenges to Survive and Opportunities to Thrive," pp. 1301–1305, Copyright 1996, with permission from Elsevier.

2. The Association of Schools of Allied Health Professions. Available at: http://www.asahp.org. Accessed March 18, 2016.

3. Lumsden G, Lumsden D. *Communicating in Groups and Teams: Sharing Leadership*. Belmont, CA: Wadsworth; 2000.

4. Spear BA, Sturdevant M, Boutelle K. The Team Approach to Treatment of Adolescents with Eating Disorders. Presentation at Food & Nutrition Conference & Expo, American Dietetic Association. October 2003.

5. Katzenbach J, Smith D. *The Wisdom of Teams*. Boston: Harvard Business School Press; 1993:45.

6. Healthy Iowans 2010 Planning Process—Roles for Key Actors. Available at: http://www.phf.org/Hptools/state/keyactors.pdf. Accessed January 28, 2004.

7. Kreitner R. *Management*, 9th ed. Boston: Houghton Mifflin; 2004.

8. Cartwright D, Zander A. *Group Dynamics: Research and Theory*, 3rd ed. New York: HarperCollins; 1968.

9. Ashforth B, Kreiner GE, Fugate M. All in a day's work: boundaries and micro role transitions. *Acad Manage Rev*. 2000;25:472–491.

10. Chatman JA, Flynn FJ. The influence of demographic heterogeneity on the emergence and consequences of cooperative norms in work teams. *Acad Manage J*. 2001;44:956–974.

11. Feldman DC. The development and enforcement of group norms. *Acad Manage Rev*. 1984;9:47–53.

12. Jewell LN, Reitz HJ. *Group Effectiveness in Organizations*. Glenview, IL: Scott, Foresman and Company; 1983:15–20.

13. Payne-Palacio J, Theis M. *Introduction to Foodservice*, 11th ed. Upper Saddle River, NJ: Prentice Hall; 2010.

14. House A, Dallinger JM, Kilgallen D. Androgyny and rhetorical sensitivity: the connection of gender and communicator style. *Commun Rep*. 1998:11;12–19.

15. Satir V. Making contact. In: Stewart J, ed. *Bridges Not Walls*, 5th ed. New York: McGraw-Hill; 1990.

16. Waldron VR, Applegate JL. Person-centered tactics during verbal disagreements: effects on student perceptions of persuasiveness and social attraction. *Commun Ed.* 1998;47:53–66.

17. Watzlawick P, Beavin JH, Jackson DD. *Pragmatics of Human Communication.* New York: Norton; 1967.

18. Thamhain HJ. Managing technologically innovative team efforts toward new product success. *J Prod Innovation Manage.* 1990;7:5–18.

19. U.S. Department of Labor. Bureau of Labor Statistics. *Occupational Outlook Handbook.* Available at: http://www.bls.gov. Accessed March 18, 2016.

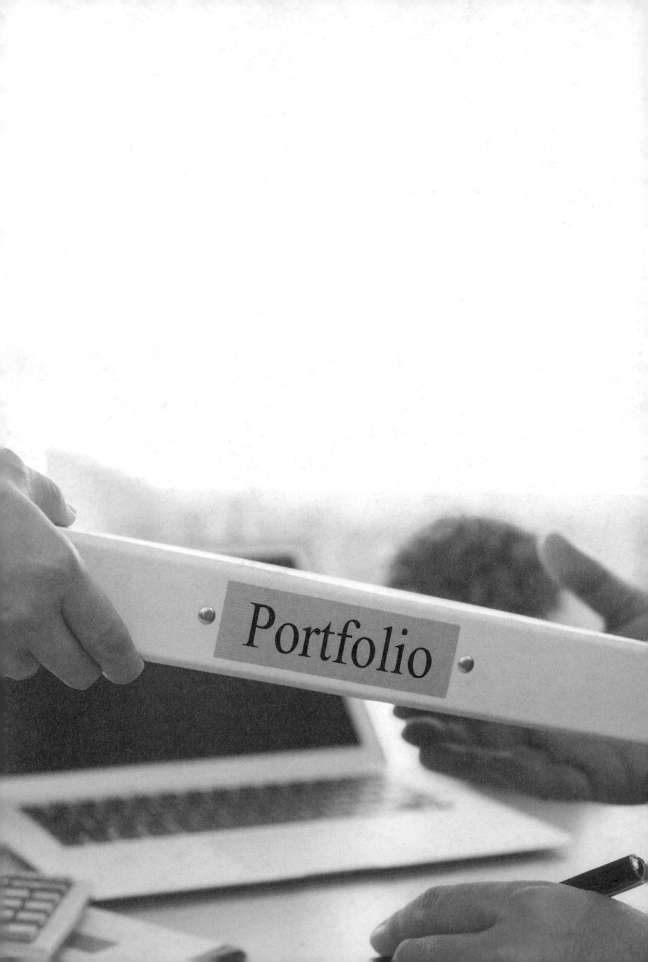

Beginning Your Path to Success in Dietetics

4

Who Are You?

Your path to success in any chosen profession begins with a bit of self-knowledge. What are your interests, strengths, and weaknesses? What are your short- and long-term goals? Where do you want to go, and how do you expect to get there? Some students are fortunate enough to have decided on their career goals by the time they begin college, but many others remain undecided.

This chapter focuses on some professional tools that will help you to answer some of the questions posed above. SWOT analysis and portfolios are useful self-assessment tools for determining your strengths, weaknesses, areas of interest, and goals. Then, a good résumé and strong interview skills and some self-marketing will help you get where you want to go.

The Portfolio

The dietetic profession's accreditation committee requires a professional development portfolio as a part of the continuing education program for registered dietitians. This portfolio is discussed in greater detail in Chapter 7. The optional portfolios discussed in this chapter—the student portfolio and the career portfolio—are of a more personal nature and will be useful to you before you reach the registration requirement stage. In fact, these portfolios are important tools for life. Always a work in progress, your portfolios should change and grow with you. New skills will be refined and demonstrated, new work experiences will be added, the number of work samples will grow and expand, and your goals and philosophy may shift and evolve to higher levels.

What is a portfolio? A *portfolio* may be defined as a coherent (not exhaustive) set of materials, including work samples and reflective statements on these samples, compiled by a person to represent his or her practice as related to desired outcomes. Some think of it as a much-expanded form of a résumé. More practically speaking, a portfolio is a collection of items organized online or in hard copy. Collecting these items throughout your college career helps you to recognize skills and abilities you possess in relation to your goals. Later, selected items from your portfolio can be placed on social media websites, such as LinkedIn, to market your qualifications for an internship or to an employer after graduation.

A portfolio is a powerful tool, not so much because of the product, but because of the process required to create it. The process takes time and thought. It is a complex, thought-provoking exercise in self-evaluation—reflection, decision making, and goal setting—that takes place over time. The product is important, too. Increasingly, selected content from the portfolio may be used in creating an online profile. This profile allows connections to be made between employers and job seekers. Online social networks represent real-world professional relationships. The profile is a unique and valuable means of communication between you and others. Potential employers, internship directors, teachers, and career counselors all may benefit from reading your profile. A sense of accomplishment, self-satisfaction, and pride is possible because your profile is a display of your individual goals, growth, and achievement, as well as a testimony to acquired knowledge and professional and personal attributes.

What Are the Purposes of a Portfolio?

Portfolios serve many purposes. The focus in this chapter is on portfolios that will initially be used for self-assessment and evaluation, to record and display professional goals, growth, and achievement. Later in your career, the professional development portfolio for maintaining registration will serve as a foundation for career-long, self-directed professional development (Figure 4-1).

Developing a portfolio in college will help you to evaluate yourself and your career decisions. Interests that are documented in your portfolio can be matched to possible careers. You can also compare the skill level displayed in your portfolio to the level needed in your chosen career. A student portfolio allows you to:

- Think about and plan your future
- Evaluate your progress
- Identify learning experiences that will help you reach your goals
- Demonstrate what you know and can do
- Learn to use a progressive tool that will be carried forward from year to year to recognize vital pieces of your personal, academic, and career development process
- Record ongoing work and accomplishments

After college graduation, a profile developed from content in your portfolio may be used to obtain an internship or job or it may follow you to graduate school. The profile allows you to demonstrate examples of work you have done and your accomplishments. An online profile also allows you to:

- Have an edge in the promotion process
- Shine in a performance review

- Distinguish yourself from the competition
- Turn a job interview into an offer
- Find the right position for you
- Create the opportunity to stand out
- Be professionally empowered
- Possess better, more authentic, more robust evidence of good practice—for reflection, discussion, and/or evaluation
- Leave a legacy to new members of the profession
- Demonstrate ability to use technology

Where Do I Start?

Your portfolio is all about making plans. The portfolio-creation process includes five steps: reflection, assessment, planning, implementation, and evaluation.

Step 1: Reflection. This first step is the most important and possibly the most difficult. The more thought you put into this step, the more rewarding your portfolio will be. The questions to ask and answer are:

- What are my strengths, weaknesses, and interests?
- What do I enjoy most in my coursework, work experiences, etc.?
- What are my short- and long-term professional and personal goals?

Answers to these questions should be written out and included in the portfolio. You may want to write a personal statement or reflective autobiography, a story of your intellectual, emotional, and spiritual growth told by the person who knows it best—you. It requires some very deep reflective thought and should work to reveal to you some new insights into who, why, where, and what you are at the present time.

Step 2: Assessment. Based on your short- and long-term goals and perceived weaknesses, what are your learning needs? Prioritize these needs based on their level of importance in reaching your goals. This step may help you to determine which classes would make good electives and what work experience would help to get you accepted to the internship of your choice.

Step 3: Planning. What is needed to accomplish your learning needs? Each learning need should relate to at least one goal, and that learning need should be accomplished with a proposed plan.

Step 4: Implementation.   Put the plan into motion. Document what you are doing or have done to accomplish your plans. A very valuable addition to a portfolio is "work in progress."

Step 5: Evaluation. Review your progress over the past few years. Evaluate what you have learned and how you have applied the new knowledge. Revise your goals as they are accomplished, writing new goals as some are achieved.

What Should I Include in My Student Portfolio?

First, keep in mind that a portfolio is representative, not comprehensive. Everything chosen should represent a significant aspect of you and/or your work. Second, because the primary purpose of the student and career

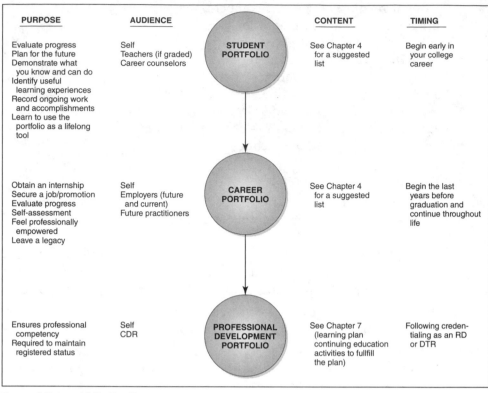

FIGURE 4–1 A portfolio timeline.

portfolios is self-assessment, every document should have a caption that leads the reader to the importance of that piece and a reflective statement. A reflective statement is simply your thoughts about the work. These thoughts might include the answers to such questions as: "What did I learn from doing it?"; "How would I do it differently the next time?"; and "Why did I receive the grade I did?"

The final point to keep in mind is that a portfolio is a work in progress and that anything included may be later deleted or added as is fitting to your professional development. Possible items to include are:

Community/Club Activities

- Certificate of participation in a program
- Evaluation written by a supervisor or other person with whom you have worked or studied
- Outline of a plan you designed to lead a program or presentation
- Pictures of members participating in an event you helped to plan
- Special notes or feedback for your help with a project
- Invitations/program/poster designed for a special event
- Records (nonconfidential) you maintained for accuracy
- Agenda describing items discussed in a committee in which you were involved

- Sketch of a layout used to determine setup of equipment and facilities for an event
- Record of the sales you achieved for fund-raising

Classroom/School Experiences
- Examples of assignments with special comments from the faculty member
- Examples of works in progress or various stages of a project
- Actual item or picture of the item created through a class project
- Report on a topic of special interest
- Outline of a memorable presentation to a class
- Transcripts of grades highlighting the classes you most enjoyed
- Certificate of completion of class or assignment
- Copy of a letter written to a person you were required to contact for a class assignment
- Pictures or souvenirs from a place to which you traveled for a field trip (**Figure 4–2**) or for study abroad
- Positive evaluation received from a faculty member or supervisor
- Summary of a research project you designed

Academic Recognition
- Letter or certificate that recognizes you as a scholarship recipient
- Letter or certificate that designates you as achieving the Dean's List

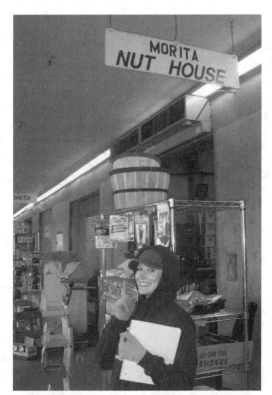

FIGURE 4–2 A dietetic student has fun on an early morning field trip to the Los Angeles Wholesale Produce Market.
Courtesy of Lari Bright

- Graduation program highlighting designation as valedictorian, salutatorian, or special honoree
- Summary of scholarly research project and/or results
- Newspaper article noting recognition of special honors
- Extracurricular activities
- Special awards for participation in an event
- Trophies/ribbons for winning or placing in a competition
- Newspaper clippings of individual or team accomplishments
- Pictures of team or individual participation in an event
- Letters or commendation from a coach, advisor, or other individuals associated with athletic achievement

Special Skills

- Examples of handouts, letters, memos, reports, charts, graphs, brochures, and so on using computer software or program languages
- Correspondence written in a foreign language or documentation of a study abroad or foreign exchange program
- Evidence of a hobby, craft, or topic of special interest, or certification of skill level such as Water Safety instructor, First Aid, or CPR
- Skill sets (groups of skills in a particular area, such as expertise with various software programs)

Work Related

- Letters of recommendation from present or former employers
- Performance evaluations
- Special recognitions from supervisor or customer for work performed
- Employee-of-the-month award
- Clippings from employee newsletter relating to you

Other

- Philosophy statement (a brief description of your beliefs about yourself and the profession)
- Academic plan of study (your plan of study that lists courses you have taken to fulfill your degree)
- Your résumé and cover letter
- Personal statement/reflective autobiography
- Career summary and goals
- List of awards and honors
- List of conferences and workshops in which you have participated
- Academic transcripts, degrees, and qualifications

The choice of what to include requires careful decision making. Asking the following questions may help:

1. What are my attributes?
2. How and what have I learned?
3. What directions for my future growth and development does my self-evaluation suggest? How can I show these in my portfolio?
4. What points have others made about me as a student? How can I show them in my portfolio?
5. What effect does my work experience have on me? How can I show this in my portfolio?

SWOT Analysis Worksheet

Internal Factors

	Your Strengths What do you do well? What do others see as your strengths? Where do you excel when compared to others?	**Your Weaknesses** What could you improve? What do others see as your weaknesses? What would make you a better practioner?	
P O S I T I V E S			**N E G A T I V E S**
	Opportunities What good opportunities are available to you? What trends could you take advantage of? Which of your strengths could you turn into opportunities?	**Threats** What trends could harm you? What competition do you face? Which of your weaknesses expose you to potential threats?	

External Factors

FIGURE 4–3 A SWOT analysis worksheet.

Turn Your Student Portfolio into a Career Portfolio

Toward the end of your college career, it is time to make some slight adjustments in the contents of your student portfolio. A SWOT analysis should be included. SWOT stands for strengths, weaknesses, opportunities, and threats (**Figure 4–3**). You can use a SWOT analysis to focus your self-assessment in order to make better decisions about your future. Understanding your strengths and weaknesses and the opportunities available to you and the threats you might face will enable you to utilize your talents, manage your weaknesses, uncover and take advantage of opportunities, and eliminate threats.

Using the worksheet, begin by writing down your strengths and weaknesses. Ask others for their opinions; be honest, objective, and realistic. Consider skills related to your career goals, teamwork, communication, and technology. Also consider your personal and social skills. For your strengths, consider the questions posed on the form. Also think about which of your achievements make you most proud. In addition to the questions on the form relating to weaknesses, what tasks do you tend to avoid because of a lack of confidence in doing them? What are your negative work habits and personality traits? Strengths and weaknesses are internal factors because they are under your control.

Opportunities and threats are external factors because you do not control them. However, you can use your strengths to take advantage of opportunities. Is there a need in the field that no one is filling? Would eliminating any of your weaknesses open up new opportunities for you? In terms of threats, what obstacles do you face in reaching your goals? How can these threats be managed or eliminated?

In addition to the SWOT analysis, the student portfolio needs to be updated and contents selected for the change in purpose and audience. As shown in **Figure 4–1**, the career portfolio is used for self-assessment as well as for obtaining a position, an internship, admission to graduate school, or a promotion. The contents of the career portfolio are a good starting point for the professional development portfolio that will be required to maintain registered status.

The Electronic Portfolio

Traditionally, portfolios have been three-ring binders or file boxes. Although this format works well for printed matter, it misses the many other ways we are able to communicate with technology. Over the past decade, most students and professionals have found that the electronic portfolio (e-portfolio) allows for a more effective way of presenting information.

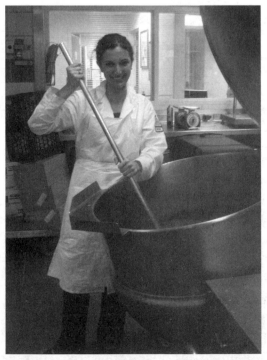

FIGURE 4–4 A dietetic intern gets hand-on experience in quantity food production.
Courtesy of Michele Coelho, RD

Digital portfolios allow the incorporation of text, images (such as that shown in Figure 4-4), diagrams, audio, video, and other multimedia elements with the benefits of minimal storage space, portability, ease of creation/updating/editing, wide accessibility, proof of technological expertise, and long shelf life. E-portfolios are not digital scrapbooks or multimedia presentations. And, although the content is useful in preparing a profile for an online social network, it is not a LinkedIn résumé.

Documents can be stored on hard drives, zip disks, or CD-ROM in many digital formats such as text documents, picture files, web pages, and digital video.

A number of websites offer tools for preparing an e-portfolio and good examples of actual e-portfolios, and others serve as hosts for web page development. Some of these sites are listed at the end of this chapter.

The Résumé

A résumé is simply a very important marketing tool that outlines your skills and experiences so that someone can see at a glance how you might fit in a position. This decision is often made in less than 30 seconds. So your résumé needs to be succinct, organized, and clearly focused on the particular purpose for which it is being used. In short, your résumé needs to stand out from the crowd and hopefully "knock the socks off" the reader!

Your résumé is also an example of your writing, communication, and organizational skills. The content, format, and style of your résumé and the accompanying cover letter are all very important details, and each is covered in the following sections.

Content

Content should **focus on relevant accomplishments and transferable competencies, not job duties and responsibilities.** A way to ensure this focus is to use project–action–results (PAR) statements when describing your school and work experiences. For example:

Project—Conducted research project on sanitation of university foodservice cutting boards.

Action—Designed and conducted the experiment.

Result—Determined best method for sanitation of cutting boards; reported results to the foodservice contractor, who implemented the method.

Where possible, quantify your experiences to convey the size or scale of projects, budgets, and/or results to make a stronger impression. Numbers, percentages, and dollars stand out in the body of a résumé. For example, rather than "Served as president of the Student Nutrition and Dietetics Association," say "Presided over 50-member Student Nutrition and Dietetics Association that resulted in five projects and nine activities (50% increase over last year)."

Include only relevant information by choosing, prioritizing, and tailoring headings and experience to the position for which you are applying. For example:

Objective—Dietetic Internship

Diet Office Experience (not Work Experience) (**Figure 4–5**)

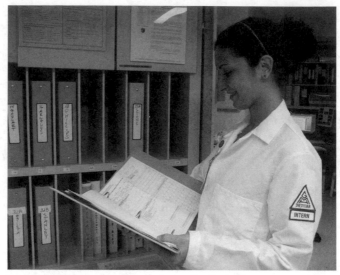

FIGURE 4–5 A dietetic intern reads a patient's chart.
Courtesy of Michele Coelho, RD

To add life to your résumé, use bulleted sentences that begin with action words like *prepared*, *presented*, *developed*, and *monitored*. A formula for building a résumé entry is as follows:

Action Verb(s) + Object/Person + to/for whom OR
of/on/from/in what OR
by/through/with what
For example:
Organized group activities in a nursing home
Answered questions on diet at campus health fair
For each job listing, ask yourself "Of which accomplishment in this position am I most proud?"

List your strengths first, where they will be most likely to be read. Rather than going into depth in any one area, use your résumé to highlight your breadth of knowledge. The interview and portfolio can then provide more detail. At all times, be honest about your skills and work experiences.

Do not include any data related to salary expectations, religious or political affiliations, geographical restrictions, age, or relationship status. Include GPA only if it is 3.0 or above.

Content headings might include any or all of the following:

- Personal Contact Information: name, address, phone, email, website
- Objective/Summary of Qualifications
- Education and Training
- Relevant Courses/Projects
- Scholarships/Awards
- Work Experience
- Relevant Skills Section
- Accomplishments/Professional Achievements
- Relevant Presentations/Publications

- Professional Affiliations
- Activities/Interests

Some experts suggest that an initial impression can be made with a résumé that begins with a profile rather than the standard objective statement. A well-written profile provides a summary of your skills and identifies your unique qualities and strengths. To write a profile, consider these questions:

Who am I?
What do I like to do?
What are my skills and abilities?
What type of work have I done in the past?
What type of work would I like to do in the future?

An example of a profile statement would be "A hard-working, energetic dietetic student who will graduate from a rigorous nutritional science program this year; experienced in hospital dietetics, undergraduate research, and working on team projects; a self-starter with a unique flair for multitasking, planning and organizing assignments, and working with people."

Format

There are basically three formats to choose from: reverse chronological, functional, and combination.

The Reverse Chronological Résumé. This format is the most commonly used, most widely accepted, most familiar to employers, and easiest to read. Work experiences are listed in chronological order starting with the most recent and working back through the years. The reverse chronological format is particularly effective when:

- You have professional experience in the field of interest
- You have held impressive job titles and/or have worked for highly regarded employers within your targeted field
- You have progressed into positions in the field with more responsibility
- You have changed jobs and fields of work frequently
- You want to change your field of work to something different from your past work experience
- You want to highlight your skills

The Functional Résumé. This format became popular in the 1970s and 1980s and is viewed skeptically by some employers. It places emphasis on your qualifications without focus on specific dates. The functional résumé summarizes your professional functions or experiences and avoids or minimizes your employment history. For example, this format would include headings such as "teaching skills," "management skills," and "patient relations skills." Each skill area is then illustrated by listing experiences that demonstrate that skill. This format is particularly effective when:

- You are a recent graduate without a lot of professional experience in the field, but you have relevant coursework and training
- You want to emphasize skills you possess that have not been used in recent work experiences

- You are changing careers (because the format outlines transferable work skills)
- You are a returning employee after an absence from the workforce or you are an older worker (because dates are minimized)

It is particularly *ineffective* when:

- You do not have a lot of time to create your résumé (it is more difficult to write)
- You want to highlight where you worked and/or the positions you have held in a particular field
- You want to highlight career growth in a particular position

The Combination Résumé. Very simply, this format uses the best components of the functional and chronological styles. The format analyzes your work strengths by area of expertise combined with a chronological listing of work experiences. It can include both chronological and skills sections. The combination résumé is the most flexible and allows for designing a very strong résumé, but it is usually longer and less widely accepted by employers. This format is particularly effective when:

- Each position you have held involves a different job description
- You have held internships or volunteer positions that relate directly to your field of interest

You should *not* consider this format when you do not have a lot of time to create your résumé.

Style

Style is critically important because résumés are typically viewed very quickly. Therefore, your résumé has very little time to make an impression. The following are some style tips that will add to the aesthetic value of your résumé:

- Use conservative, plain, and easy-to-read fonts; do not use more than two font styles and do not use smaller than 9-point font. A reasonable size is between 9 and 12 point. Sans serif fonts like Arial or Verdana come out much clearer than Times New Roman in faxes.
- Be concise! Keep it to one page in length. In most cases, not everything will fit. This will require cutting and pasting the content down to the most relevant and most impressive for the position in question. The résumé should match the job description.
- Do not crowd too much on a page, make good use of white space, emphasize what is most important, and allow at least a 1-inch margin on all sides.
- Use bold, italics, capitalization, and underlining minimally and consistently to emphasize what is most important. Use simple bullets to separate duties and skills.
- Balance material on the page so that it is pleasing to the eye. Put the most important information about one-third from the top, do not hide it at the bottom.
- Use high-quality bond paper in white, off-white (beige or ivory), or gray; these are the easiest to read. Résumés, cover letters, and envelopes should all match.

- Print on one side of the paper only.
- Be sure the copy has no blurring, stray marks, or faint letters (a laser printer is preferred for clarity and neatness).
- Avoid phony or stilted language, word repetition, unnecessary words or phrases, and the use of any pronouns, particularly "I."
- Avoid the use of acronyms and abbreviations that the reader may not understand.
- Proofread carefully and then proofread again. Use the spell and grammar check tool on your computer.
- Have several people critique your résumé—someone to proofread, someone familiar with the field, and someone unfamiliar with the field.

The Cover Letter

A résumé should always be accompanied by a cover letter. The cover letter will be read before the résumé and, like the résumé, the average time spent reading the letter will be about 20 seconds. Many of the same principles discussed in the section on résumé writing apply to writing the cover letter. It is important to be concise and clear. The letter is a reader's first impression of your writing and organizational skills. The paper used should match your résumé paper; content, formatting, and style all count.

The first paragraph should talk about how you heard about the position and some of your strengths that relate to the job. Do some research on the company and discuss why this company/organization appeals to you. In the second paragraph, briefly describe your qualifications, skills, and accomplishments. Do not just repeat your résumé. This is your chance to point out your outstanding qualities, to direct the reader's attention to any parts of your résumé that are most relevant, to explain any part of your work history that needs clarification, and to show your personality. Your résumé will fill in the details. In the third paragraph, you should relate yourself to the organization: why you would be a good fit and what you could bring to the company. The last paragraph should contain the fact that your résumé is enclosed, a request for an interview appointment, and how and when the employer may easily contact you. Here are some tips for the letter:

- Be sure to personalize your cover letter. Find out the name of the person who will be reviewing your résumé; never use clichés such as "Dear Sir or Madam" or "To Whom It May Concern." If you cannot get a name, use "Dear Internship Director" or "Dear Employer."
- Be specific, clear, and to the point; keep it to one page.
- Proofread the letter very carefully; double and triple check for spelling and grammatical errors.
- Follow standard business letter format.
- Keep copies.
- Do not forget to sign the letter.
- Be yourself.

A skillful, unique cover letter is the best way to demonstrate your intelligence and personality and get you an invitation for an interview.

The Interview

Your cover letter and résumé worked, and you have an appointment for an interview. The interview process can make even the most self-confident person nervous because so much rides on this face-to-face encounter. Even though some nervous energy is positive, too much may be detrimental to your success. The best way to overcome the sense of dread and foreboding is to prepare, prepare, prepare and to look and sound confident during the interview.

The chances are that your interview will last from 15 seconds to 30 minutes. The interviewer will often make his or her decision about you in the first few seconds or minutes of the interview. The other 25 to 29.75 minutes will be a courtesy to you if you have already been screened out. If, however, the results of the first impression are favorable, the interview will last the full half-hour or longer. Achieving this result requires knowing what's important. Employers and graduate schools are looking for some basic qualities: communication skills, appearance, personality, ability to think, energy level, and leadership potential. Be prepared to demonstrate your possession of each of these qualities.

Keep in mind that an interview is a two-way street. Just as the interviewer wants to know if you are right for the position, you want to know if the position is right for you. The interview is your opportunity to find out about the position, the organization, and the culture, and how these might fit into your career goals.

Basics of Interviewing

Some key points to keep in mind on the day of your interview include:

- Be certain of the date, time, and exact place of the interview (including directions and parking).
- Arrive at least 10 to 15 minutes early. Relax, get a drink of water, check your appearance, collect your thoughts, and visualize a positive interview.
- Carry a pen and notepad to make notes of important points. You might also want to jot down the questions you want to ask. Ask permission to take notes.
- Come equipped with extra copies of your résumé, lists of references, and a pen that is readily accessible.
- Wait for the interviewer to offer to shake hands, stand straight, make eye contact, and use a firm grip—neither brute force nor limp.
- Do not smoke or chew gum.
- Wait until the interviewer sits or invites you to sit before doing so.

Basic Preparations for the Interview

Before the day of your interview:

- Research the school/company/organization using the Internet, printed materials, and conversations with faculty, alumni, students, employees, and others.

- Think through your responses to questions according to the type of interview: direct question/answer, indirect ("tell me about yourself?"), or group or board/committee (several interviews and/or several interviewers). Lists of hundreds of typical interview questions are available at the websites listed at the end of the chapter. It is a good idea to prepare answers to some of the most frequently asked questions. Do not memorize the answers, or they will sound too rehearsed.
- Think of questions you want to ask. Your questions will reflect your interest, intelligence, personality, thought processes, and curiosity.
- Assess what you have to offer and be prepared to express that.

The Interview Itself

During the interview, you have to communicate your motivation, experience, and skills as well as project your personality. In order to do this:

- Be sincere, courteous, tactful, and enthusiastic.
- Be thorough but concise in your answers. Don't talk too much. Telling the interviewer more than he/she needs to know may be a fatal mistake and "rambling on" indicates lack of preparation.
- Keep the interviewer's attention by being articulate and varying the tone, volume, and tempo of your voice. Speak clearly and audibly.
- Control the content of the interview. Interviewers will ask specific questions. Your responses should directly address the questions and can then smoothly transition to an area or subject that you want to talk more about.
- Display interest in the interview and treat every question as important.
- Listen carefully to the questions or comments. When they are vague, ask for clarification: "Do I understand your question to be...?" Let the interviewer know you heard what is being said.
- Use the "pause-to-think method" (taking your time to organize your thoughts in your mind before responding) when you need to regroup or organize thoughts.
- Avoid negative comments about fellow students, former employers, coworkers, and professors of classes in which your grades were lower.
- Be prepared to respond to questions about your weaknesses as well as your strengths.
- Respond tactfully to questions about your personal life whether or not you understand their relevance to your motivation, qualifications, or goals.
- Be yourself and do not attempt to second-guess what the interviewer would like to hear.
- Do not be intimidated by your competition. Think positively.
- Be prepared for a sophisticated, professional interview technique. If he or she is an experienced interviewer, you will be prepared. If not, you have the advantage.
- Be honest and consistent in your responses.

- Distinguish between questions that call for fact versus those that call for opinion.
- Be confident. Believe in yourself. But avoid cockiness. There is a fine line between confidence, professionalism, and modesty. Overconfidence is as bad as, if not worse than, being too reserved.
- Observe the interviewer and copy his or her demeanor, style, and pace. Don't be too familiar. This is a business meeting and not about making a new friend.
- Maintain a comfortable level of eye contact without staring. If you are being interviewed by a group of people, make sure to address all of them with your eyes.
- Be prepared to ask questions. To break a long silence, say, "May I ask a question about...?" Have some questions ready to ask, but avoid questions about salary and benefits at the first interview. The best questions are follow-ups to what you are being asked, requesting additional information. This demonstrates your interest in the company and allows you to decide if it is the right place for you.
- Use appropriate language, avoiding inappropriate slang and references to age, race, religion, politics, and sexual orientation.
- To redirect the interview to you, ask a question related to something you would be interested in doing (e.g., "Would there be an opportunity during the internship to work on a research project with you or other faculty members, and, if so, when would that be possible?")
- Don't appear desperate. A candidate who interviews with the "please, please, hire me" attitude appears less than confident. Remember the 3 C's: cool, calm, and confident.
- Review your past interviews to improve your techniques for future interviews.
- Encourage yourself.

Closing the Interview

When the interviewer brings the interview to a close, first thank him or her for meeting with you. This should be followed by a question regarding when a decision will be made or what the process is from here.

Tips for Nervousness

It is natural to feel some nervousness before an interview. Some ways to help alleviate this feeling are:

- Get enough sleep before the interview.
- Concentrate on the questions and your responses.
- Take deep breaths and use the pause-to-think method.
- Do not worry about complex questions. If you do not understand a question, do not hesitate to ask for clarification.
- Before and between interviews and in private, practice relaxation techniques by closing your eyes and relaxing one part of your body at a time.

Additional Guidelines

First impressions are important during the interview process. A few additional guidelines for creating a positive first impression are listed below.

- Look neat and clean and dress somewhat conservatively.

Men

Wear a suit or sport jacket with color-coordinated trousers.
The color should be neutral—dark blue, black, or gray is best. Wear a tie.
Shoes should be leather—clean and polished—black is best.
Make sure your nails are trimmed and clean.
Head and facial hair should be neatly trimmed.
Cover any tattoos.

Women

Wear a classic suit or a simple dress with a jacket.
Appropriate colors are navy blue, black, dark green, dark red, burgundy, or gray.
Avoid wearing clothes that are tight, revealing, or trendy.
Fingernails should be trimmed and, if painted, should be in a conservative color.
Hair should be done appropriately—avoid wild hairdos.
Avoid gaudy jewelry and limit pierced jewelry to ears only. Cover any tattoos.

- Do not wear fragrances, because many people are allergic. Bathing with good-quality bath soap with a mild scent and using an unscented antiperspirant will cover any nervous perspiration.
- Be aware of your posture and avoid distracting "mannerisms," such as foot tapping and touching your hair.
- Remember to turn off your cell phone and/or pager during the interview.
- Write a handwritten thank-you note within 48 hours after each interview. Thank the interviewer for his or her time, again mention your qualifications, and affirm your desire for the position. Do not use email for this note.

Summary

Success in your chosen career in large part depends on knowing yourself. This knowledge allows you to capitalize on your strengths, determine what you want to do and where you want to go, and continuously make improvements in areas that may need strengthening. Beginning to create a student portfolio at the start of your college career is a powerful way to attain this self-knowledge. Toward the end of your college career, turn your student portfolio into a career portfolio. The portfolio creation process requires self-evaluation, reflection, decision making, and goal setting. It has the potential to be a vehicle for career-long professional development and a source of unrivaled personal satisfaction.

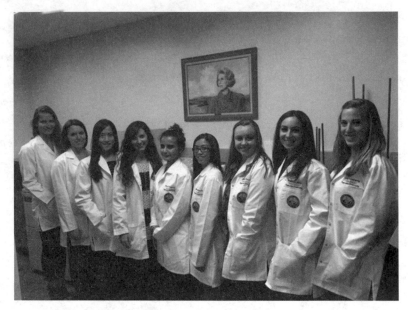

FIGURE 4–6 A graduating class of proud dietetic interns.
Courtesy of Susan Helm, PhD, RDN, Pepperdine University.

A portfolio may also be used as a communication tool to present you and your work to others by turning it into an e-portfolio and online profile. While you are a student, your portfolio may be required for evaluative purposes and may actually be graded. When you are a professional, your online material is a valuable expansion of your résumé in the interview or job review process. It can be used to generate conversation about your abilities and interests and things you have accomplished and, perhaps most important, provide actual proof of work you have done (**Figure 4–6**).

If your portfolio is a comprehensive view of who you are, your résumé is a snapshot. It is a one- to two-page document that summarizes you and your experiences to attract the attention of potential graduate school directors, employers, colleagues, and others. Because it is the first impression you give a company, presentation and organization of the résumé are critical. Careful attention should be paid to content, format, and style in creating a résumé that will get you an interview.

A cover letter should always accompany a résumé. It is the cover letter that will be read first and very quickly. For these reasons, the cover letter should be clear, concise, personalized, carefully proofread, aesthetically pleasing, and dynamic.

Once an interview is secured, it should be approached with careful preparation and handled professionally. Preparation before the interview includes knowing and understanding your own accomplishments and goals, researching the organization that is interviewing you, thinking of the questions you need to ask, thinking of the answers to questions you may be asked, and being prepared with your portfolio, résumé, and references.

Handling the interview professionally requires that you are well groomed and dressed appropriately, display good manners, treat everyone with courtesy, stay relaxed and focused, and be yourself.

With the self-evaluation provided by a portfolio, a sharp résumé, strong interviewing skills, and online self-marketing tools, you are on your way to career success in your chosen field of endeavor.

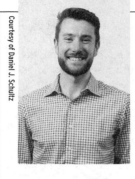

Courtesy of Daniel J. Schultz

Profile of a Professional

Daniel J. Schultz, MS, RDN

Project Administrator at ChildObesity180
Friedman School of Nutrition Science and Policy, Tufts University, Boston, Massachusetts

Education:
BS in Human Biology with an emphasis on Nutritional Sciences and Dietetics, University of Wisconsin–Green Bay, Green Bay, Wisconsin
MS in Community Health with an emphasis on Sustainable Food Systems and Nutrition, Montana State University, Bozeman, Montana

How did you first hear about dietetics and decide to become a Registered Dietitian?
The catalyst for my career in dietetics began as a child when I personally dealt with the issue of childhood obesity. After I made significant behavior changes and improved my health as a young adult, I became highly interested in learning as much as possible about nutrition. The tipping point to make it my career occurred during my freshman year of college, when my friend Max told me about the professional field of nutrition and dietetics. I was beyond excited and started to pursue the registered dietitian credential after switching universities and majors.

What was your route to registration?
After taking 2 years off to serve with the AmeriCorps Program, FoodCorps, I enrolled at Montana State University in a pilot coordinated masters and internship program.

Where did you complete your supervised practice experience?
I completed my supervised practice through the Montana Dietetic Internship. I worked in the communities of Bozeman, Helena, Missoula, Livingston, and Polson, Montana.

How have you been involved professionally?
While in Iowa serving with FoodCorps, I became involved with the professional organization of Iowa State University Extension and completed the process to become a Master Gardener. Additionally, I'm currently a member of the Academy of Nutrition and Dietetics and their Hunger and Environmental Nutrition dietetic practice group.

What honors or awards have you received?
- Marie Moebus Dietetic Internship Scholarship Recipient
- FoodCorps Food Talk Presenter on Childhood Obesity
- Iowa American Heart Association Heart Story Recipient
- University of Wisconsin–Green Bay Chancellor's Medallion
- Tri-Beta Biology Honor Society
- Half marathon finisher medals and one full marathon finisher medal

Briefly describe your career path in dietetics. What are you doing now?
After my nutrition coursework at the University of Wisconsin–Green Bay, I served 2 years with the national service program, FoodCorps, where I coordinated nutrition education and helped underserved students and families get excited about healthy food. My service involved helping the Des Moines Public School District with school gardens, local sourcing, after-school cooking programs, and in-classroom Supplemental Nutrition Assistance Program (SNAP) nutrition education.

Additionally, my career has involved writing nutrition articles for websites like Livestrong.com, eHow, and SFGate Healthy Living. My coordinated graduate program at Montana State University focused on the nutritional implications of government food assistance programs such as SNAP and the Special Supplemental Nutrition Program for Women, Infants, and Children (WIC). I also researched the integration of nutrition and agriculture into the field of dietetics and the unique sustainable food systems concentration for the Montana Dietetic Internship. During my dietetic internship, I also completed an internship at the U.S. Department of Agriculture's Center for Nutrition Policy and Promotion.

On a national and local level, I have also been an advocate for a healthy food environment and prevention of childhood obesity. My work has been featured on the CBS Evening News, *The New York Times* Blog, Ecocentric.com, *The Des Moines Register*, and Iowa Public Radio. Currently, I share my food policy and nutrition research as a contributor for the *Huffington Post*, Healthy Living, Impact, Political and Food columns.

In my current position as a project administrator at ChildObesity180, I help schools implement walking and running programs. This position involves a lot of community engagement, technical assistance, and strategic communication. In Boston alone, we are helping over 8,000 students and 60 schools improve students' health and academic performance through physical activity.

What excites you about dietetics and the future of our profession?
I'm excited that it is finally food and nutrition's time in the spotlight. Never before has there been such a national interest on the question of what we all should be eating for health. Although, misinformation still abounds around nutrition, I feel that registered dietitians can build off of this momentum and begin to lead the way with education and environmental changes to make the healthy option the easy and preferred choice.

How is teamwork important to you in your position? How have you been involved in team projects?
For my current position, I work with the Active Schools Acceleration Project team at ChildObesity180. From meetings, traveling to conferences, and project implementation development, teamwork is the important fabric that makes our work a success.

What words of wisdom do you have for future dietetics professionals?
My current advice to any future dietetic professional is to take a systems approach to your work. As important as it is to make an impact with individual counseling sessions, as practitioners, everyone must be aware of the social determinants of health and policies in place that impact the client's health outcomes and food choices. As future registered dietitians, you have the power and knowledge to help advocate for policies and system changes that create a culture of health in your community.

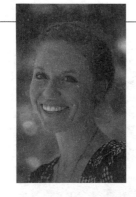

Profile of a Professional

Jessica Wrye, RD
Registered Dietitian and Bilingual Health Educator at OLE Health, Napa California.

How did you first hear about dietetics and decide to become a Registered Dietitian?
I decided to study nutrition while volunteering at a soup kitchen throughout my high school years. After seeing how crucial food is in people's daily lives, I knew I wanted to learn more about how to best meet people's needs. Once I was plugged into college nutrition courses, I was exposed to the dietetic's career path and RD certification process.

What was your route to registration (internship, coordinated program, pre-planned experience, etc.)?

My journey has been quite the roller coaster! The first time I applied to dietetic internship programs I was not accepted. Even though it felt like failure at the time, it has turned out to be the best thing that could have happened to me. Not only did this teach me grit, but it gave me the unique opportunity to work as a DTR (dietetic technician, registered) at the Atascadero State Mental Hospital. It was during this difficult job that I discovered my passion for nutrition as it relates to mental health. At the next round of DI applications, I was accepted into my top choice. Already having professional experience in dietetics made me more than prepared to overcome the challenges of a dietetic internship.

At what college or university did you receive your entry-level education? What was your degree in? (Nutrition? Dietetics?)

I received my undergraduate degree in Nutrition & Dietetics from California Polytechnic State University and graduated *cum laude*.

Where did you complete your supervised practice experience?

My 10 month dietetic internship program was based out of Tri-County Health Department in Denver, Colorado. In addition to working at the largest public health department in Colorado, I was exposed to diverse dietetic settings around the metro area. Some of the highlights included Denver Health Medical Center (level 1 trauma medical center), Colorado Children's Hospital, University of CO Anschutz Medical Center (research rotation), and Aurora Public School District (food service management overseeing 53 schools).

Do you have advanced degree(s)? If so in what and from where? (What was your degree in? Nutrition? Food Systems Management? Business?)

I do not currently have any advanced degrees. However, I do plan to work towards a Master of Public Health so I can better learn how to plan effective community programs.

Briefly describe your career path in dietetics. What are you doing now?

I received my RD certification in October 2015 and have since been working at a nonprofit community clinic that serves over 25,000 patients, practices an integrated care model, and partners with other community organizations. I work with a team of dedicated medical professionals to help patients prevent/manage chronic diseases by individual appointments in Spanish or English for medical nutrition therapy. Part of this work also includes teaching nutrition education classes among those suffering from severe mental illness and recovering from substance abuse. Finally, I am on a wellness team partnering with the Napa County Health & Human Services that is designing a care-network program for those with coexisting chronic diseases and mental disorders.

What excites you about dietetics and the future of our profession?

It is always growing/evolving! There are so many different health disparities where RDs can play a bigger role in joining multidisciplinary teams to better meet the needs of the community. One of those areas is managing and preventing chronic disease among those with mental health disorders, a widely underserved population.

Why/how is teamwork important to you in your position? How have you been involved in team projects?

We cannot meet the true needs of an individual or community without teamwork. I believe in taking a holistic approach, which means looking at all aspects surrounding a problem and listening to one another's strengths and expertise in a multidisciplinary setting. In team projects, I enjoy playing the facilitator role by asking lots of questions and reminding the team of the big picture.

What words of wisdom do you have for future dietetics professionals?

First, there is no one cookie-cutter path to becoming a RD and you never know what gems you might learn from failure. Second, do not be afraid to step outside the box and challenge the status quo. As the profession of dietetics continues to grow/evolve with new research, we need unique pioneers that ask lots of questions and never stop learning!

Suggested Activities

1. Ask a classmate or friend to list five adjectives that describe you. Try to use these in writing your personal statement.

2. Print out some of the lists of potential interview questions from the websites listed at the end of this chapter. Think of answers you might give if asked any of these questions.

3. Role play actual interviews with classmates, including direct, indirect, and illegal questions that might be asked. (It is illegal to ask any question that might be discriminatory because of race, religion, sex, age, marital status, or national origin.)

4. Need more help with your résumé? Free templates are available online. Search the Internet to find one that is appropriate for you.

5. Read the article "8 Questions to Ask in an Interview for an Internship" at http://www.monster.com/career-advice/article/8-questions-ask-internship-interview.

6. Want to see a sample of a good résumé? Visit your college placement center and ask to see résumé samples.

7. Either working alone or in teams in class, select a position or specific job (e.g., intern, graduate school candidate, part-time diet office clerk) for which you might apply, and write a list of questions that you might ask during the interview.

8. As you begin to develop your portfolio, give some thought to the following questions:

   - What kind of person do I want to become (desirable characteristics and rejected characteristics)? What can I do to achieve this?
   - What are the characteristics that I want and do not want in my career? What can I do to achieve them?
   - What role do I want in the community and professional organizations? What can I do to achieve this?
   - What kind of family life is important to me?
   - What level and variety of activity do I want?
   - How much effort am I willing to exert to achieve my objectives? Summarize the answers to these questions into a list of objectives and action plans.

9. List, in order, five personal characteristics that others seem to appreciate most in you. How did each one develop? How could you use each one to greater advantage? List, in order, five personal characteristics that seem to result in difficulties when dealing with others. How did each one develop? What, if anything, has been or could be done about each one? What other setting might tolerate, if not value, the characteristics most?

10. Identify the major areas of your work or student responsibilities. Rate yourself in each area compared with others in your age and work groups (lowest 25%, middle 50%, next 15%, top 10%). What have you done to improve your performance, and what were the results? What are the biggest obstacles to your improving your work or academic performance? What have you done about each, and what were the results?

Selected Websites

- http://www.collegegrad.com—Résumé, cover letter, and interviewing information
- http://ehe.osu.edu/career-services—Information on interviewing, résumés, and cover letters
- http://gecd.mit.edu/jobs/find/prepare/resume—Site offers tips on preparing résumés and cover letters
- http://www.monster.com/career-advice/—Job listings, résumé postings, help with tools for job searches
- http://www.linkedin.com—World's largest business-oriented social media network
- http://www.webs.com—Website building with suggested themes and templates
- http://www.weebly.com—Site offers templates and tips for building your own website
- http://www.wix.com—Create your own website; templates and tips are offered
- http://www.freewebspace.net—Website hosting and tools for building

Suggested Readings

Portfolios

Barrett H. Using "free" online tools for e-portfolio development. Available at: http://www.electronicportfolios.com. Accessed November 9, 2015.

Barrett H. Electronic portfolios. Available at: http://www.electronicportfolios.com. Accessed November 9, 2015.

Electronic portfolios: Students, teachers, and life-long learners. Available at: http://educscapes.com. Accessed November 9, 2015.

Frank JS. Electronic portfolios in hospitality, foodservice management and dietetic education. Presentation at Foodservice Management Education Council, March 9, 2015.

Houston CA, Venter-Barkley J. Dietetic student portfolio assessment: it's "elementary" using the moSTEP framework as a model. *DEP Line.* 2003;24(Winter):5–11.

Langevin DD. Professional portfolio assessment: a tangible documentation of achievement of the competencies. *DEP Line* 2003;24(Winter):12–13.

Payne-Palacio J. *A Portfolio Primer: An Introduction to Profession Portfolios and the Issues Associated with Their Use.* Malibu, CA: Pepperdine University; 2004.

Quinn JE. Use of authentic assessment through student portfolios. *DEP Line.* 2003;24(Winter):1–9.

Rood R, Martin Mildenhall A. "Portfolio" assignment, Utah State University Dietetic Internship. *DEP Line.* 2003;24(Winter):4–9.

University of Lethbridge, Canada. A guide to the development of professional portfolios. Available at: http://www.uleth.ca/education/sites/education/files/portfolioguide.pdf. Accessed April 8, 2012.

Williams AG, Hall KJ, Shadix K, Stokes DM. *Creating Your Career Portfolio*. Upper Saddle River, NJ: Prentice Hall; 2005.

SWOT Analysis

Personal SWOT Analysis. Available at: http://www.mindtools.com. Accessed March 18, 2016.

SWOT Analysis. Available at: http://www.valuebasedmanagement.net/methods_swot_analysis.html. Accessed March 18, 2016.

SWOT Template. Available at: http://www.whatmakesagoodleader.com/swot_template.html. Accessed March18, 2016.

Résumés/Cover Letters

Allen JG. *The Resume Makeover*, 2nd ed. New York: John Wiley & Sons; 2001.

American Dietetic Association. Resume writing tips for entry-level RDs and DTRs. *J Am Diet Assoc*. 2007;107(4):S10.

American Dietetic Association. Sample resume of someone with management-level experience in the dietetics profession. *J Am Diet Assoc*. 2007;107(4):S8–S9.

American Dietetic Association. Sample resume of student or first-time job seeker in the dietetics profession. *J Am Diet Assoc*. 2007;107(4):S7.

Beatty R. *The Resume Kit*. New York: John Wiley & Sons; 2000.

Block J. *101 More Best Resumes*. New York: McGraw Hill; 1999.

CampusAccess.com. Resume and cover letters. Available at: http://www.campusaccess.com/careers/resumes.html. Accessed March 18, 2016.

CollegeGrad.com. Everything you need to know about cover letters. Available at: http://www.collegegrad.com/coverletters. Accessed March 18, 2016.

CollegeGrad.com. Quickstart resumes. Available at: http://www.collegegrad.com/resumes/quickstart/index.shtml. Accessed March 18, 2016.

Massachusetts Institute of Technology. Five steps to writing a great resume. Available at: https://gecd.mit.edu/jobs-and-internships/resumes-cvs-cover-letters-and-linkedin/resumes. Accessed March 18, 2016.

Ohio State University. Resume writing and cover letters. Available at: http://ccss.osu.edu/undergraduates/job-internship-search-strategies/resume-writing-and-cover-letters/. Accessed March 18, 2016.

Resumes. Available at: http://www.eresumes.com. Accessed November 10, 2015.

vos Savant M. Ask Marilyn. *Los Angeles Times, Parade Magazine* 2004;January 11:16.

Interviewing

American Dietetic Association. Interviewing tips for entry-level registered dietitians. *J Am Diet Assoc.* 2007;107(4):S13.

CampusAccess.com. Interviews. Available at: http://www.campusaccess.com /careers/interviews.html. Accessed March 18, 2016.

Massachusetts Institute of Technology. Ace the interview. Available at: https://gecd.mit.edu/jobs-and-internships/interviews-and-offers/interviewing. Accessed March 18, 2016.

Ohio State University. Interviewing skills. Available at: http://ccss.osu.edu /undergraduates/job-internship-search-strategies/interviewing-skills/. Accessed March 18, 2016.

Ten tips to boost your interview skills. Available at: http://www.monster .com.Accessed November 10, 2015.

PART III

Preparing for Practice

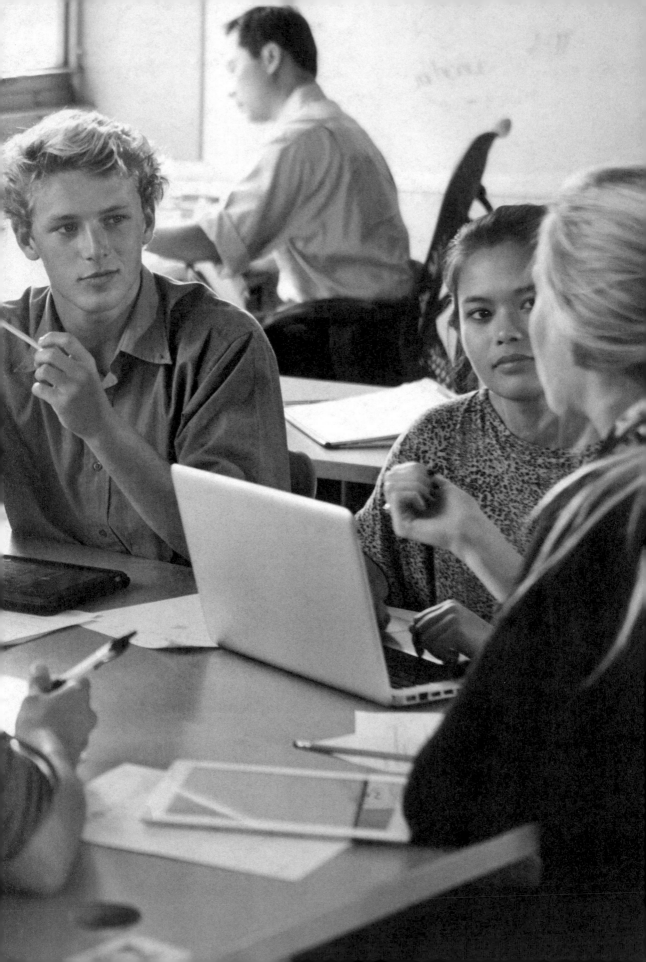

Dietetics Education and Training

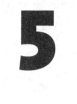

Have I Got a Plan for You!

One of the first actions of the fledgling American Dietetic Association (ADA) was the establishment of a teaching section to provide guidance in the education and training of dietitians.[1] From the very earliest days of the profession, academic education has been paired with hands-on, "real-world" experience.[2] The 1927 issue of the *Journal of the American Dietetic Association* published the first "Standardization of Courses for Student Dietitians in Hospitals," as proposed by the section on education of the ADA. Entrance requirements for the hospital-based training program required the dietetic student to be 21 years of age and have a minimum of a bachelor's degree with a major in foods and nutrition from a college or university of "recognized rank."[3]

Many of the subsequent journal articles through the years focused on the hospital portion of the student dietitian's training more than on the academic preparation that preceded the hands-on experience. Early on, the challenge of preparing individuals for the real world of dietetics practice was evident. Mary W. Northrop, a dietitian at Montefiore Hospital in New York City, stated in 1929, "We must take the college girl who comes to us and make her into a professional woman; that six months is too short a time in which to accomplish so complete a metamorphosis is obvious. It seems probable that we shall be forced either to increase the length of our courses or to demand that the colleges send us more mature and competent students."[4]

Times have certainly changed since Ms. Northrop wrote that article! Yes, the dietetics profession is still predominately female, but education programs have advanced beyond "taking the college girl and making her into a professional woman"! Men are joining our profession in increasing numbers; so to the men reading this chapter, please don't despair. Dietetics education programs strive to make professionals of both genders!

The suggested course of study found in the December 1940 issue of the *Journal of the American Dietetic Association* may look vaguely familiar to today's dietetics majors. General chemistry, organic chemistry, and biochemistry were required, as well as human anatomy and physiology, psychology, sociology, economics, educational psychology, food preparation, advanced courses in nutrition, and numerous courses in quantity cookery, organization, and management.[5]

Since 1947, the educational requirements for entry-level dietitians have been revised several times. The last version—"Eligibility Requirements and Education Standards"—was published in 2012. Standards are published individually for each kind of dietetics education program: Nutrition and Dietetics Technician Education Programs, Dietitian Education Programs, Didactic Programs in Nutrition and Dietetics, Internship Programs in Nutrition and Dietetics, Foreign Dietitian Education Programs, as well as Guidelines for Advanced-Practice Residencies. The current academic requirements for each program may be found on the Academy of Nutrition and Dietetics website www.eatright.org.[6]

For many years, the only way to become a dietitian was to obtain a bachelor's of science (BS) degree that met the organization's academic requirements, followed by completion of a post-baccalaureate dietetic internship. In 1962, however, the first Coordinated Program (CP) in Dietetics was developed, which combined the required internship with the academic program. The student's hands-on experiences were coordinated with what was being discussed in the classroom, with the goal of making the combined learning experience even more meaningful. Through the CP, a student could theoretically fulfill the academic and internship requirements in 4 years rather than 5.

In the early 1970s, the need for dietetic support personnel led to the development of associate degree programs for dietetic technicians. These programs combined a 2-year associate degree with 450 hours of hands-on experience.

The Certified Dietary Manager, Certified Food Protection Professional (CDM, CFPP) is a credential awarded by the Association of Nutrition and Foodservice Professionals (ANFP). Individuals with this credential act in a supervisory capacity in food production management and sanitation and, in some practice settings, monitor nutritional status in consultation with a Registered Dietitian Nutritionist. Find out more information about the CDM, CFPP credential at http://www.anfponline.org/become-a-cdm/cdm-cfpp-credential.

The Accreditation Council for Education in Nutrition and Dietetics

The Accreditation Council for Education in Nutrition and Dietetics (ACEND) is recognized as the accrediting agency for associate-degree Nutrition and Dietetics Technician Programs, baccalaureate-level Didactic Program in Dietetics (DPDs), baccalaureate and graduate-level CPs, and post-baccalaureate Dietetic Internships (DIs). According to the Academy of Nutrition and Dietetics website:

> *ACEND serves the public by establishing and enforcing eligibility requirements and accreditation standards that ensure the quality and continued improvement of nutrition and dietetics education*

*programs that reflect the evolving practice of dietetics. ACEND
defines educational quality as the ability to prepare graduates with
the foundation knowledge, skills and/or competencies for current
dietetics practice and lifelong learning.*[7]

ACEND has a 15-member board.[8] In addition, a group of peer reviewers
with expertise in dietetics education and practice is appointed by ACEND, as
needed, to visit and evaluate programs and make recommendations on accreditation. Currently, 136 of these peer reviewers have been trained to evaluate
and assist dietetics education programs in the accreditation process.[9] ACEND
functions as the governing unit and grants final accreditation awards.

ACEND's Standards and the Accreditation Process

ACEND outlines five standards that must be met by every dietetic education
program:

- **Standards on Program Eligibility for ACEND Accreditation.** These
  standards relate to program sponsorship, organization, financial
  resources, and leadership. The goal is to make sure the program has
  a structure in place that will ensure success in achieving program
  excellence.
- **Standards on Program Planning and Outcomes Assessment.** These
  standards are designed to ensure that the dietetic education program
  has a clearly stated mission, goals, and objectives. The program must
  have an assessment process in place with appropriate outcome measures that allows for ongoing program improvement and determining if
  the program's goals and objectives have been met.
- **Standards on Curriculum and Student Learning Objectives.** These standards help to make sure the program's curriculum gives students the
  proper foundation in the areas that form the basis of dietetics practice
  (biomedical, nutritional, behavioral, managerial, and clinical sciences).
  The content and sequencing of the curriculum and the type of practice
  experiences must be appropriate to prepare graduates for successful
  careers. Methods of promoting student learning and development of
  lifelong learning skills and the assessments to measure these must be
  documented.
- **Standards on Program Staff and Resources.** These standards help to
  ensure that the dietetics program has fair policies and procedures and
  capabilities to attract, develop, and retain well-qualified faculty and
  staff so that the program's goals and objectives can be achieved. The
  program must also demonstrate that it has adequate and appropriate
  facilities and resources to offer a high-quality program.
- **Standards on Students.** These standards help to ensure that the program
  provides adequate resources as well as fair policies and procedures
  to support students and their progression and personal/professional
  development.[6]

Before a dietetic program can begin accepting students, the program's
director and faculty members must undertake an in-depth review process
known as a *self-study*. The process for conducting a self-study is outlined in

ACEND's "Candidacy for Accreditation" document.[6] The self-study document outlines, in detail, how the dietetic program meets the ACEND standards. The written self-study document is then forwarded to ACEND and selected peer reviewers.

In previous years, this written self-study was all that was required for certain types of dietetics programs. If peer reviewers deemed that the program's self-study document adequately showed how the program was meeting the standards, the program was "approved" by the accrediting body. However, ACEND now requires that all dietetic education programs be accredited. **Accreditation** means that the program not only writes a self-study document, but the peer reviewers also visit the program to verify that what was written in the self-study document is actually occurring. These site visits are opportunities for the program faculty to interact with the peer reviewers as they work together to ensure that the program's graduates are well prepared and ready for dietetics practice. The site visits also show students, parents, administrators, and others that the dietetic education program meets the high standards set by ACEND.

A dietetic education program that offers only the coursework necessary to meet the accreditation standards is called a Didactic Program in Dietetics (DPD). A dietetic education program that offers only the supervised practice experiences necessary to meet ACEND standards is called a DI. Coordinated Programs, International Dietitian Education Programs (IDEs), Foreign Dietitian Education Programs (FDEs), and Dietetic Technician Programs provide both the academic component and the required supervised practice experience within the degree program. Thus, the self-study document for these programs must outline how both the academic and supervised practice requirements are met for their respective types of programs.

Grievance/Complaint Procedure

If any individual, such as a student, faculty member, dietetics practitioner, or member of the public, has a complaint about an accredited dietetics education program, he or she may submit a complaint or grievance to ACEND. ACEND has established a process for reviewing complaints to fulfill its public responsibility for ensuring the quality and integrity of the educational programs that it accredits. However, ACEND makes it clear that "it will not intervene on behalf of individuals or act as a court of appeal for individuals in matters of admissions, appointment, promotion, or dismissal of faculty or students. It will act only upon a signed allegation that the program may not be in compliance with the accreditation standards or policies." The procedure for complaints against programs can be found on the Academy's website at www.eatright.org.[10]

The Steps to Becoming a Registered Dietitian Nutritionist or Nutrition and Dietetics Technician, Registered

A Registered Dietitian Nutritionist (RDN) is a food and nutrition expert who has met the minimum academic and professional requirements to qualify for the RDN credential. Many RDNs deliver medical nutrition therapy in hospitals, health maintenance organizations (HMOs), private practice, or other healthcare facilities. In addition, a large number of RDNs work in community and public health settings, in academia, and in research. RDNs also work in facets of the food industry, such as school foodservice, college and university foodservice, healthcare foodservice, food manufacturing and sales, corporate wellness programs, and sports nutrition.[11]

A Nutrition and Dietetic Technician, Registered (NDTR) is a food and nutrition practitioner who has completed at least a 2-year associate's degree at a U.S. regionally accredited university or college, required coursework, and at least 450 hours of supervised practice accredited by ACEND or at least a bachelor's degree at a U.S. regionally accredited university or college and required coursework for a DPD. A DPD graduate who has had no supervised practice during his or her educational program may want to obtain supervised practice experience to better prepare for the credentialing examination and the job market. In addition, the individual must pass a national NDTR examination administered by the Commission on Dietetic Registration (CDR) and complete continuing professional educational requirements to maintain registration. The majority of NDTRs work with RDNs in a variety of employment settings, including health care (assisting RDNs in providing medical nutrition therapy), in hospitals, HMOs, clinics, or other healthcare facilities. In addition, a large number of NDTRs work in community and public health settings, such as school or day care centers, correctional facilities, weight management clinics, and Women, Infants, and Children (WIC) programs.[12]

The steps in the preparation for dietetics practice are academic preparation, supervised practice, confirmation of academic preparation by verification from the program director, confirmation of appropriate supervised practice (if required) by verification from the program director, and credentialing by passing the Registration Examination for Nutrition and Dietetics Technicians or the Registration Examination for Registered Dietitian Nutritionists. These steps apply whether you wish to become a NDTR or an RDN.

To Become a NDTR, You Must . . .

There are two options by which one may become a NDTR:

1. Complete a Nutrition and Dietetics Technician Program that is accredited by ACEND of the Academy of Nutrition and Dietetics that includes 450 hours of supervised practice experience in various community programs and healthcare-related and foodservice facilities and complete at least a 2-year associate's degree at a U.S. regionally accredited college or university (**Figure 5–1A**).

OR

2. a. Complete coursework in an ACEND-accredited didactic program or coordinated program in dietetics and complete at least a bachelor's degree at a U.S. regionally accredited college or university.

   b. After completing the degree and dietetics coursework, pass the national dietetic technician examination by the CDR. See the CDR website at http://www.cdrnet.org for further information about the examination (**Figure 5–1B**).

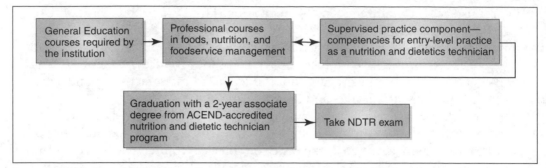

FIGURE 5–1A Nutrition and Dietetics Technician Education Option 1. A specific grade-point average or other criteria may be required for the student to participate in supervised practice activities. Check with the program director for specific program requirements.

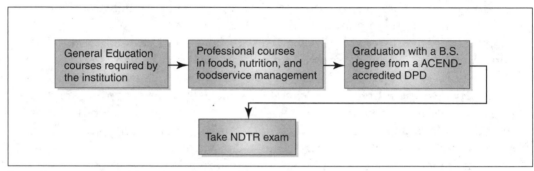

FIGURE 5–1B Nutrition and Dietetics Technician Education Option 2.

c. Complete continuing professional education requirements to maintain the NDTR credential. See the CDR website at http://www.cdrnet.org for further information about continuing professional education requirements.

To Become an RDN, You Must . . .

1. Complete the minimum of a baccalaureate degree in an accredited DPD or CP that meets ACEND's "Core Knowledge for the RDN." Completion of the academic requirements must be verified with a signed Verification Statement from the program director.
2. Complete a minimum of 1,200 hours of supervised practice experience within an accredited CP or accredited DI that meets ACEND's "Core Competencies for the RDN." Completion of the supervised practice requirements must be verified with a signed Verification Statement from the program director.
3. Successfully complete the national Registration Examination for Dietitian Nutritionists (**Figures 5–2** and **5–3**).

If You Already Have a Baccalaureate Degree, You Must . . .

If you already have the minimum of a baccalaureate degree in any area and wish to become a NDTR or an RDN, you must first have your transcripts

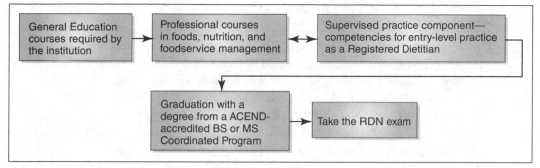

Figure 5–2 Coordinated Program in Dietetics (may culminate in a baccalaureate or a master's degree). A separate application process for admission to the supervised practice component of the program is typically required. Every supervised practice program has its own admissions criteria and application process. Check with the program director for further information.

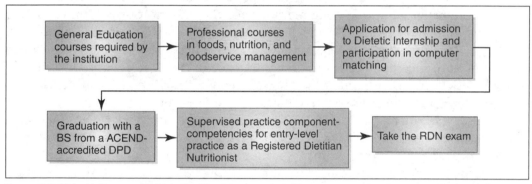

Figure 5–3 Didactic Program in Dietetics Plus Dietetic Internship. Every supervised practice program has its own admission criteria and application process. Dietetic internships may have an optional or required graduate education component. Submission of GRE scores and/or acceptance to graduate school may be part of the application process. Check with the program director for further information.

Note: If you already have the minimum of a baccalaureate degree in any area and wish to pursue becoming a Nutrition and Dietetics Technician, Registered or a Registered Dietitian Nutritionist, you must first have your transcripts evaluated to ascertain what additional courses you will need to take to meet the current ACEND knowledge requirements. This evaluation must be completed by the program director at the ACEND-accredited academic program to which you are seeking admission. Earning an additional degree in dietetics may or may not be required, depending on the policies of the institution. Once the appropriate academic requirements have been completed, you may then pursue application to the appropriate supervised practice experience program and finally sit for the credentialing examination.

evaluated to ascertain what additional courses you will need to take to meet the current ACEND "Core Knowledge for the RDN." This evaluation must be completed by the program director at the ACEND-accredited academic program to which you are seeking admission. Earning an additional degree in dietetics may or may not be required, depending on the institution's policies. Once the appropriate academic requirements have been completed, you may then pursue application to the appropriate supervised practice experience program and then sit for the credentialing examination.

The Academy website includes additional resources that depict the various education pathways for dietetics students. These can be found in "The Basics for Students" portion of the Academy of Nutrition and Dietetics website at www.eatright.org.[13]

The Academic Experience

The academic preparation to become a dietitian may be obtained in either an accredited DPD or CP. Nutrition and Dietetics Technician students obtain their academic preparation in an accredited Nutrition and Dietetics Technician Program or an accredited DPD program. The dietetics curriculum may be slightly different at different universities, because each school has unique strengths and resources. Graduates of DPDs are eligible to apply for post-baccalaureate supervised practice programs to meet the Academy's requirements. CP graduates meet both the academic and supervised practice requirements in their degree programs and are eligible to sit for the Registration Examination for Dietitian Nutritionists upon completion of their degree (**Figure 5–2**). Likewise, graduates of an accredited Nutrition and Dietetics Technician Program meet both the academic and supervised practice requirements in their associate's degree program and are eligible to sit for the Registration Examination for Nutrition and Dietetics Technicians upon completion of their program.

What knowledge, skills, and abilities are necessary for dietetics professionals to meet the needs of the marketplace in the days ahead? How should dietetics education respond to the Academy's strategic plan and the identified emerging dietetics-related issues of obesity, aging, complementary care, dietary supplements, safety of the food supply, and genetic engineering? Dietetics educators face many challenges in building the best curriculum to answer these and many other questions. Each dietetics education program builds the curriculum to prepare students for the dynamic future of dietetics. Because communication skills are so critical for success in dietetics practice, courses in composition and speech are included. Dietetics practice is grounded in science; thus, courses in biology, anatomy and physiology, microbiology, and chemistry are part of a student's program of study. Having a foundation in these subjects enables students to understand concepts in their professional foods and nutrition courses.

Courses in psychology and sociology help future dietitians understand how people think and act, either individually or in groups. Courses in business, such as economics, marketing, and accounting, prepare students for the managerial and business aspects of dietetics practice, which must be understood no matter what area of dietetics a person might pursue. Because the public eats so many meals away from home in restaurants, fast-food operations, cafeterias, and so on, future dietitians need to understand how food is prepared and served to the public. Basic foods courses help dietetics students learn food science principles and food preparation for the home; however, quantity foods courses prepare students to work with clients in the institutional or commercial foodservice arenas. Courses in normal nutrition, public health nutrition, medical nutrition therapy, and nutritional counseling prepare students for nutritional assessment, diagnosis, and intervention with individuals and groups.

Because the profession of dietetics holds so many options and opportunities, the choice of electives in a student's educational program can build skills in areas that may be useful in the future. Being able to speak another language will be increasingly important as our society becomes more and more diverse. Going beyond the basics of word processing and spreadsheet development to learn more about technology can open doors and enhance the application of technology to dietetics practice. Taking additional courses in business, such as finance, organizational behavior, or entrepreneurship, can prepare students for cutting-edge opportunities. Coursework in gerontology can prepare students to work with the rapidly growing elderly segment of our society. The list of possible elective courses is extensive. The curricula of dietetic education programs will continue to evolve as the profession of dietetics continues to change and grow.

Students who are participating in a coordinated program in dietetics or a Nutrition and Dietetics Technician Program will have courses that have a supervised practice component. A dietetic education program with a supervised practice component (Nutrition and Dietetics Technician Program, CP, or DI) also must include a concentration area as part of the curriculum. The concentration area doesn't mean that the student becomes a specialist in the area, but rather allows the student to gain some additional depth in a particular aspect of dietetics practice. The concentration area(s) is chosen on the basis of the mission, goals, resources, and expected learning outcomes developed by the program.

The Academy website lists 223 ACEND-accredited DPDs. DPDs are available in the District of Columbia, Puerto Rico, and all states. Some states have numerous accredited DPDs: Texas has 16, California has 16, and Illinois has 11. Currently, 56 CPs, 42 Nutrition and Dietetics Technician Programs, and 247 dietetic internships are accredited by ACEND. The Academy website lists programs by state and distinguishes those programs that offer distance education, those that have course credit transfer agreements, and those that offer graduate degrees.[14] CPs, DIs, and Nutrition and Dietetics Technician Programs—all of which meet ACEND's supervised practice requirement—are discussed in greater detail in the next chapter.

Distance Education in Dietetics

Distance education is defined as "planned learning that normally occurs in a different place from teaching and as a result requires special techniques of course design, special instructional techniques, and special methods of communication by electronic and other technology, as well as special organizational and administrative arrangements."[15] Distance education is a growing phenomenon in education today, and the world of dietetics education is no exception. At present, four DPDs offer the complete baccalaureate degree in dietetics online. Three CPs, 20 DIs, and 5 Nutrition and Dietetics Technician Programs are available in a distance education format.[14] Many programs offer some coursework by distance education. Because of the increasing interest of the public in food and nutrition issues, more and more individuals are interested in the profession of dietetics as a career. Because of the flexibility and asynchronous nature of distance education, this format particularly meets the needs of students who are working in full-time jobs and/or have family responsibilities that may prevent them from taking classes during the day or relocating to a university with a dietetics program.

Many modes of distance education delivery are possible. Although print-based correspondence courses are still available, many universities are using a wide variety of technologies to bring the classroom into the student's home or workplace. Online courses, CD courses, videotaped courses, audioconferencing, videoconferencing, or combinations of these formats may be used. Some distance programs offer their complete curriculum in a distance format, both general education and professional courses. Other schools may offer degree-completion programs, in which students take the first 2 years of general education courses at a local community college or other institution and then enroll in the distance education program to complete the "professional" foods, nutrition, and foodservice management courses.

Distance education technology may also be used by dietetics programs to offer flexibility in their on-campus courses. Traditional "face-to-face" classes may also use a web support page as a means of posting the course syllabus, maintaining an online grade book, offering a course message board or "chat room" options, and posting other information. On-campus students may use distance technology to interact with off-campus counterparts. Moreover, distance education technology is being used to provide continuing education to credentialed dietetics professionals. Online graduate programs are beginning to appear, and continuing education short courses are increasing. Educational technology is here to stay!

Is distance education right for you? The pros and cons of distance education have been widely discussed. Positive factors include:

- Convenience—the course may be as close as your computer with an Internet connection.
- Flexibility—you can attend class on your schedule because the material is available 24 hours a day, 7 days a week.
- Availability—more and more universities are providing distance education coursework.
- Accessibility—you can work anywhere you have computer access.
- Self-directed—you have more control over the learning environment and can set your own pace or schedule.
- Cost—taking courses online is usually cheaper than incurring moving costs and other expenses involved in relocating to a traditional university setting.

Negative aspects of distance learning include:

- No campus atmosphere—part of the traditional college experience is actually being on campus, soaking up the atmosphere, and experiencing traditional college life.
- Limited social interaction—you do interact with classmates and instructors via email, chat rooms, and discussion groups, but you miss some of the social interaction that is often part of the traditional on-campus experience.
- No face-to-face time with the instructor—the amount of one-on-one interaction you have with the course instructor varies from course to course and university to university. However, if you are the kind of student who likes personal attention from your instructor, distance education may not be for you.

- Making time—if you are a procrastinator or if you need a push to complete your work, you may have a difficult time with the self-discipline necessary to work independently in distance classes.
- Requires new skills and technology—if you are "technophobic" and are uncomfortable with computers and technology, then online education may be a struggle for you, at least in the beginning.
- Expense—you may need specific computer hardware or software to participate in the distance education program, which may lead to additional expense.
- Test taking—you may need to go to a specific location for proctored examinations or to make other special arrangements for taking tests.[16]

When making decisions about a distance education course or program, use the same decision-making steps you would take in deciding about which traditional school to attend:

- Check out the program thoroughly. How long has it been in existence? Are the university and program accredited by the appropriate accrediting agencies? How many people are enrolled in the program, and how many have graduated? What is the success rate of this program's graduates in obtaining a post-baccalaureate dietetic internship? In passing the RDN or NDTR exam?
- Talk to other people. Ask if you can interact with current students or graduates of the program. See what they have to say about the quality of the courses and the level of interaction with faculty. What kind of response time did they experience between the time they posed a question and the time they got an answer? What kind of feedback and assistance did they get from faculty?
- Visit by email, phone, or in person, if possible, with the program director. Talk to that person about the program, its philosophy, and its goals. What kinds of resources will be made available to you as a distance education student? As a distance education student, how are you made to feel a part of the university and the program? Do your best to ascertain if you are a good fit for the program.

Distance education is the wave of the future in entry-level education and continuing education. Whether you experience distance education technology in a few courses or whether your whole degree program is obtained in this way, you are probably getting a first taste of the educational delivery system of the future.

Service Learning in Dietetics

Another type of pedagogy that is becoming more and more common in today's dietetics education programs is service learning. Service learning is defined as "a teaching method that combines explicit academic learning objectives with community service."[17] Nothing reinforces abstract, theoretical concepts discussed in class like the opportunity to try out those concepts in a real-life situation benefiting the student's community. Service learning can make textbook theories come alive for students.

According to Chabot and Holben,[18] service learning has numerous advantages for dietetic students. You can acquire both social skills and academic knowledge while enhancing your ability to work with diverse individuals and groups. Assignments have more meaning when they are part of a service learning project rather than a "dry" academic exercise. Participating in service learning can help meet real needs and help you feel more connected to your community. Service learning fosters citizenship, personal development, social responsibility, interpersonal skills, and tolerance. Finally, service learning can provide you with an opportunity for career exploration and can lead employment opportunities. Chabot and Holben[18] give examples of service learning placements, including working at local soup kitchens and homeless shelters; volunteering with Meals-on-Wheels programs; working with groups such as the American Red Cross, the American Cancer Society, the American Heart Association, and other similar groups; and participating with Habitat for Humanity, Big Brothers/Big Sisters, and local hospice organizations. The list goes on and on. Assisting professionals who work in such organizations and seeing what they do and how they do it provides valuable learning experiences for future dietetics professionals.

Verification of Academic Requirements

Upon successful completion of the academic program, the student is issued a Verification Statement. This form is a legal document and should be treated as such. This document, bearing the original signature of the program director, verifies that the student has successfully completed the academic portion of entry-level requirements. Students completing a DPD and a post-baccalaureate supervised practice program will have two Verification Statements; students completing a CP or a Nutrition and Dietetics Technician Program will have only one. These statements must be presented when the student changes from student to active membership in the Academy or when the graduate applies for a license to practice dietetics in a state that has licensure for dietetics professionals.

Building a Career Portfolio

According to Williams and colleagues,[19] a portfolio is "a collection of materials designed to show your work or competencies in a specific area." Many dietetic education programs require each student to compile a portfolio during his or her academic program that showcases the student's skill and abilities. Increasingly, portfolios are developed and accessed online. Examples of materials that may be found in a portfolio include the following:

- A statement of originality (indicating that the contents belong to you and asking people viewing the contents to keep the information confidential)
- A statement of your work philosophy
- Career goals
- A brief biography

- Your résumé
- Skill areas, including work samples, letters of recommendation, and skill sets (checklists of critical skills related to the area)
- Works in progress
- Certifications, diplomas, degrees, scholarships, and awards
- Professional memberships/affiliations and certifications
- Academic plan of study
- Supervised practice plans
- Publications
- Faculty and employer biographies
- References

Building and maintaining a career portfolio is an ongoing process. As you move through your schooling and supervised practice experiences, you will continually be adding new material to your portfolio and removing material that may no longer be relevant. It is not a good idea to upload actual copies of your projects or assignments as this may make it possible for other individuals to plagiarize your work.

As you enter dietetics as a practicing professional, you will create and maintain your career portfolio as part of the CDR credentialing process. Chapter 7 in this text provides more detailed information about the professional development portfolio. Because the portfolio process will be an ongoing part of your life as a dietetics professional, it makes sense for you to start learning about portfolios and building your own now as a student (see also Chapter 4).

Graduate Education

After many years of discussion, data collection and analysis, and lively debate, in February 2015, ACEND recommended that a master's degree be the level of educational preparation for entry-level, generalist, RDNs. ACEND is in the process of developing new standards for master's degree–level programs and will be releasing these for public comment in 2016. Once revisions are made and the new standards and competencies are finalized, ACEND plans to release them in 2017 for voluntary adoption by pilot dietetic education programs. Outcomes data on graduates of these pilot programs will be collected and analyzed before ACEND makes a decision about implementation of the recommended future model for all programs. ACEND will work with the CDR to define the credentialing options for those completing these new degree programs. The goal is for the transition to the master's degree for entry-level to be accomplished by 2024.

This move to requiring a master's degree for entry into the profession is not without considerable controversy. Will increased respect be accorded to RDNs with a master's degree? Will RDNs with a master's degree see salary increases? Will requiring a graduate degree integrated with supervised practice help lessen the backlog of qualified students who have not been able to secure an internship? Will requiring a graduate degree make increased diversity in dietetics an even more challenging goal? There are also concerns about requiring the master's degree adding time and cost to the already long career journey to enter the dietetics profession, leading to burnout and increased levels of student debt as one starts their dietetics career.

The Academy of Nutrition and Dietetics's "2015 Compensation & Benefits Survey of the Dietetics Profession" revealed that 48% of all RDNs already hold a master's degree, indicating that members of the profession value advanced education.[20] The report noted, "Education beyond the bachelor's degree is clearly associated with wage gains." However, data show that at the 50th percentile of salaries reported, RDNs with a master's degree reported making $31.48 per hour, whereas those with a bachelor's degree earned $28.85 per hour, a difference of only $2.63 per hour. While 46% of survey respondents reported receiving some form of employer assistance for professional development (such as tuition reimbursement), such a benefit will not be quite as helpful if new RDNs have to have the master's degree *before* sitting for the credentialing exam and gaining employment. Dietetics is one of the several health professions considering a graduate degree for entry to the profession. For example, physical therapy now requires a practice doctorate to enter the profession. Occupational therapy is also considering a practice doctorate requirement for entry into their profession, with a target date of 2025 (see http://www.aota.org/aboutaota/get-involved/bod/otd-faqs.aspx). Students considering entrance into dietetics should keep informed on the topic of required graduate education as they progress in their education.

You might think that the decision of whether to attend graduate school is something far in the future. As the requirement for a graduate degree moves toward reality, the subject of graduate school takes on considerable importance and relevance for students *now*. Students should keep this in mind even as they are pursuing their undergraduate education. Remember that academic performance at the undergraduate level is a major criterion for admission to graduate school. Typically, a 3.0 grade point average (GPA) at the undergraduate level is required for a person to be admitted to a graduate program. The applicant may also be required to take a graduate school admissions test, such as the Graduate Records Examination (GRE) or the Graduate Management Admissions Test (GMAT). A review of the applicant's undergraduate GPA, performance on a standardized admissions test, letters of recommendation from professors and/or employers, and a clear and concise statement of goals for graduate study often make up the graduate school admission process.

There are various opinions about whether a student should go straight from an undergraduate program directly into a graduate program or whether the student should work a few years before pursuing graduate study. This is another point of controversy in the decision to require the graduate degree for entry into the profession. The graduate school experience is different from the undergraduate program. Graduate classes are often smaller than undergraduate ones, and classes tend to be more "discussion driven." A student coming straight from his or her baccalaureate program into a graduate program without having much "real-world" experience may find him- or herself somewhat at a loss to contribute to class discussions in the same way as others who have had more work experience in the field. Work experience also allows an individual to hone his or her interests and may be the source of questions that might be answered in a master's thesis or doctoral dissertation!

Currently, a growing number of post-baccalaureate dietetic internships offer the new graduate the opportunity to pursue a master's degree concurrently with obtaining the required DI experience. Many students find this opportunity exciting, and see the master's degree/internship combination as a chance to further their education in a more in-depth and focused way while meeting the dietetics supervised practice requirements.

Master's degrees may be earned in any number of areas, including the following:

- MPH—Master of Public Health
- MBA—Master of Business Administration
- MS—Master of Science (in a variety of subjects)
- MEd—Master of Education

Currently, CDR has indicated that the master's degree can be in any area. However, students will still need to meet the Core Knowledge competencies, whether in their undergraduate program or as part of their master's degree program. As pilot programs and outcomes analyses unfold in the next few years, many of the questions and controversies will be answered and clarified.

Most master's degree programs require 30 to 36 credit hours beyond the baccalaureate degree. A master's program may be research oriented, with the student completing both coursework and a research project. The student writes a thesis that incorporates a review of pertinent literature; a description of the research idea/problem, methodology, and data analysis; a description of the findings; conclusions drawn; and recommendations for future research. A master's program may also be non-thesis, meaning that instead of doing a research project the student takes additional coursework. At the conclusion of the program of study, students may be asked to pass a comprehensive written and oral examination over their academic program of study.

Graduate study at the doctoral level also may be completed in a variety of disciplines:

- PhD—Doctor of Philosophy (in a wide variety of disciplines)
- EdD—Doctor of Education
- DSc—Doctor of Science
- DBA—Doctor of Business Administration
- JD—Doctor of Jurisprudence or Doctor of Law
- MD—Doctor of Medicine

Most doctoral programs are considered approximately 90 credit hours of study beyond the baccalaureate degree, about 30 credits hours of which may be research. Doctoral degrees involve advanced coursework, completion of a major research endeavor, and the writing and defense of a dissertation. Individuals who complete doctoral degrees often teach in colleges and universities, work as researchers in higher education or in industry, or become chief executive officers of organizations.

The benefits of advanced study are both tangible and intangible. Many people pursue advanced study because of their intrinsic drive to learn and grow. Having an advanced degree may enhance a person's status and enable the person to earn a higher salary or be promoted to new levels of responsibility and authority. Graduate education should also help the individual to understand the research process and to develop teamwork, critical thinking, problem solving, communication, and other skills that can make him or her more marketable and successful in his or her professional endeavors. The Academy website (www.eatright.org) has a list of graduate programs in areas that may be of interest to dietetics professionals.[21]

Summary

Preparation for entry into the profession of dietetics encompasses both prescribed academic preparation and supervised hands-on experience. Both of these components are carefully structured and monitored by the Academy through its Accreditation Council for Education in Nutrition and Dietetics. Ongoing practice audits form the basis for the "Core Knowledge" and "Core Competency" statements used to guide the development of both academic curricula and supervised practice experiences. A complete listing of all accredited dietetic education programs of every type can be found on the Academy website, www.eatright.org.[22]

The challenge facing the Academy and dietetic educators is to keep educational preparation on the cutting edge of professional practice, ensuring that current students will be prepared for the exciting future that awaits them as dietetic technicians and registered dietitians. The most important focus must be on the development of critical-thinking and problem-solving skills, so that future dietitians know how to think, rather than what to think. Future dietitians must be prepared to take responsibility for their own continued professional development, because information about food and nutrition issues is expanding at an exponential rate. By learning how to learn, the dietitian student will be ready for an exciting future in dietetics.

Suggested Activities

1. Find out about the history of your dietetics program. When did the program begin? How many people have graduated from your program? What are some of those graduates doing now?
2. Interview a dietitian in your area. Ask the dietitian the following questions:
   a. How did you learn about the profession of dietetics?
   b. What kind of dietetics education program did you go through?
   c. What was your first dietetics position?
   d. What other dietetics positions have you held?
   e. Describe your current job and its responsibilities.
   f. What skills do you believe are necessary for successful dietetics practice?
   g. What do you like best about being a dietitian or dietetic technician?

3. Access the listing of dietetic education programs on the Academy website (www.eatright.org). Are there other dietetics education programs in your state? In a neighboring state? If so, where are they? What kinds of programs are offered? Contact some of the students in these programs and network with them!

4. Select two dietetics programs other than your own. Go to the websites of each program and read about them. Compare the curriculum and experiences of each program with the program in which you are enrolled. What are the commonalities? What are the differences?

5. Review the "Core Knowledge" and "Core Competency" statements for the type of dietetic education program in which you are enrolled. This listing may be found on the Academy website (www.eatright.org). Compare these requirements with your dietetics curriculum to see how your curriculum helps prepare you to meet these requirements.

6. Compare the "Core Knowledge" and "Core Competency" statements for Nutrition and Dietetics Technicians and RDNs. Explain how the education and training for NDTRs complement the training of the RDN and enable the two professionals to work together in a supportive relationship.

7. Check out dietetics programs that have a distance education option. These may be found on the Academy website (www.eatright.org) under the listing of all accredited programs. How do these programs work? What are the pros and cons of this educational approach? Contact a distance dietetics program and interview one of their students to learn more about the experience.

Selected Websites

- www.eatrightpro.org/resources/career/professional-development/advanced-degrees—A search engine at the Academy Student Center for advanced degrees.
- www.eatrightpro.org/resources/career/become-an-rdn-or-dtr—A section at the Academy of Nutrition and Dietetics site about becoming an RDN or DTR.
- www.eatrightacend.org/ACEND/content.aspx?id=6442485469—Area of the ACEND website to learn more about the accreditation process and standards for the various types of dietetic education programs.
- www.eatrightacend.org/ACEND/content.aspx?id=6442485414—This site contains a listing of all ACEND-accredited dietetic education programs.
- www.eatrightacend.org/ACEND/content.aspx?id=6442485390—Visit this site to learn about the procedures for complaints against an accredited program.

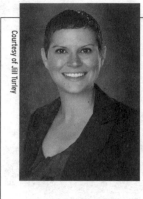

Profile of a Professional
Jill Turley, MS, RD, LS, SNS

National Nutrition Advisor
Alliance for a Healthier Generation (https://www
.healthiergeneration.org/)
Education:
BS in Human Nutrition, Oklahoma State University, Stillwater,
Oklahoma
MS in Human Nutrition, Oklahoma State University, Stillwater,
Oklahoma

How did you first hear about dietetics and decide to become a Registered Dietitian?
I was working at the Bureau for Social Research at Oklahoma State University, where
we conducted telephone interviews to collect survey information. One study I worked
on was with former dietetics graduates. I became very interested in the subject and
began researching the program at Oklahoma State University (OSU) and career
opportunities in the field.

What was your route to registration?
I completed my internship through OSU.

Where did you complete your supervised practice experience?
I completed my internship at OSU in various institutions around the state of
Oklahoma. My foodservice management rotation was completed at St. Mary's Hospi-
tal in Enid, Oklahoma. My clinical rotation was completed at Integris Baptist Medical
Center in Oklahoma City, Oklahoma.

**What are some examples of professional involvement at the local, state, or national
level at the American Dietetic Association/Academy of Nutrition and Dietetics or
other professional associations?**
Academy of Nutrition and Dietetics; School Nutrition Association.
Past Affiliations and Positions Held:

- Oklahoma Academy of Nutrition and Dietetics (2009–2011 Senior Editor, ODA
  Nutrition Manual; 2010–2011 Public Relations Chair; 2006–2008 Board of Directors)
- North Central District Dietetic Association (2010–2011 Area Representative; 2008–
  2009 Area Representative; 2007–2008 President)
- Dietitians in Business and Communications (2007–2010 Contributing Editor, DBC
  Dimensions)

What honors or awards have you received?
2012 Emerging Dietetic Leader, Oklahoma Academy of Nutrition and Dietetics; 2011
Rising Star Alumni Award, College of Human Sciences, Oklahoma State University;
2005 Outstanding Dietetic Intern, Oklahoma Academy of Nutrition and Dietetics.

Briefly describe your career path in dietetics. What are you doing now?
I spent 6 years in the food industry immediately after my internship. There, I was
responsible for nutrient analysis of the company's products; I then moved into advis-
ing our product development and marketing teams. I worked primarily in the K-12
channel during that time, where I helped develop lower sodium products, as well as

other products, to help foodservice directors meet the school nutrition standards. I assisted marketing with bringing products to market, and I supported the K-12 sales force. I also provided nutrition-related training and professional development to foodservice directors around the country.

In my current role at the Alliance for a Healthier Generation, I provide strategic input regarding food and nutrition issues for the Alliance's Healthy Schools Program and Healthy Out-of-School Time initiative. I am responsible for assessing the professional development needs of schools and sites and creating and delivering appropriate in-person and virtual training materials and workshops, specifically around competitive foods and beverages, school nutrition services, and healthy eating. I assist schools as they implement the USDA's Smart Snacks in School nutrition standards. I develop and enhance nutrition-related tools and resources for schools and out-of-school time sites, including the Alliance's online food tools. I also maintain relationships with various national stakeholders.

What excites you about dietetics and the future of our profession?
The possibilities are endless. We are a profession focused not only on nutrition, but also on food. And it's exciting to see more intersection with actual food, whether through opportunities in the food industry or at a community and household level. I am a foodie at heart, and I hope to see more of a culture shift to focusing on real, simple food and incorporating that into lifelong healthy habits. Our profession is in a unique position to facilitate that shift.

How is teamwork important to you in your position? How have you been involved in team projects?
I could not get my job done without my amazing team! Our team does a lot of training and resource development for various groups, and it is so helpful to have people to bounce ideas around with. Brainstorming with others is such a valuable benefit to teamwork. I also believe it is vital to develop trusting relationships with your team members so you feel comfortable letting go of tasks or projects when needed. In our team, not only are we in constant development mode, but we also travel a great deal. Having a group I can rely on when responsibilities need to shift based on deadlines or travel schedules is priceless. I work with my immediate team on training and resource development, but I also work across teams at the Alliance on broader strategies and actions for our organization related to nutrition. Additionally, I had the invaluable experience in my previous job to work across many teams as I followed a product from conception to roll-out.

What words of wisdom do you have for future dietetics professionals?
Get in the kitchen and cook. Know your way around food. Know how to translate complex nutrition science into practical, actionable steps. Meet people where they are, which often is not nose deep in clinical nutrition science. We have to be able to transform that science into messages that resonate with people. Break it down and show them how it fits in their day-to-day life. And day to day, food is generally in the kitchen! We can tell people all day long that asparagus is healthy. But what if they don't know what to *do* with asparagus? Teach them what to do with it. Don't be afraid to play with your food so you can show others how to do the same!

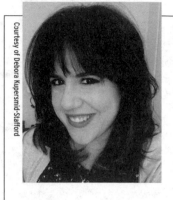

Profile of a Professional

Debora Kupersmid-Stafford, MS, RD, CDN

Registered Dietitian Nutritionist
Urban Health Plan, Inc., Bronx, New York

Adjunct Lecturer
Queens College, City University of New York, New York,
New York

Education:
BS in Nutrition and Exercise Sciences, Queens College, City
University of New York, Flushing, New York
MS in Nutrition and Exercise Physiology, Teachers College at
Columbia University, New York, New York

How did you first hear about dietetics and decide to become a Registered Dietitian?
I first heard about the dietetics programs when I was completing my undergraduate degree in Nutrition and Exercise Sciences at Queens College, but because I was not sure in what path I wanted to take with my career I did not pursue it. As I started the graduate program at Teachers College, Columbia University, I realized that dietetics was the field for me and going through the internship program was vital. Teachers College Nutrition community nutrition, medical nutrition therapy, and nutrition education classes were very engaging and exciting, so as I was taking the classes, I realized this was my passion: to teach and share my knowledge and to help people live better, healthier lives.

What was your route to registration (internship, coordinated program, preplanned experience, etc.)?
Once I decided to pursue the path to become a Registered Dietitian, I spoke with my advisors in school to determine which classes I needed to take. The last year and a half of my graduate-level education I was full time in school, working part time as a teaching assistant at Queens College, City University of New York, and taking the undergraduate courses required to enter a dietetic internship program. I took classes such as microbiology, foodservice management, and food science in three different universities, two online and one in person. It was a busy year indeed!

Based on what I felt I wanted to do in the field, I applied to the Teachers College, Columbia University Dietetic Internship program. It was a bold move to only apply to one program in this very competitive field, but I was sure that this internship would be the best suited for my career goals. A few months later, I got in! I completed the 11-month program, which included seven rotations—three in clinical sites, three in community sites, and one in foodservice—and then we had options for elective rotations, in which I returned to one clinical and one community site.

Where did you complete your supervised practice experience?
For my supervised practice experience, I had seven rotations (three clinical, three community based, and one in foodservice) in New York City and The Bronx.

Clinical:

1. Mary Manning Walsh Nursing Home. In this rotation, I performed supervised nutrition assessments, interventions, and evaluations of short-term/rehabilitation as well as long-term patients. I also participated in health initiatives such as health fairs.
2. Naomie Berrie Diabetes Center. In this rotation, I shadowed RDs and nurse practitioners who provided education both in English and Spanish to type I and type II diabetics as well as patients with gestational diabetes. I also developed multiple handouts and diabetic-friendly recipes, in English and Spanish, to provide nutrition education to patients.

3. Manhattan Physician's Group. In this rotation, I shadowed and eventually provided nutritional counseling to a variety of pediatric, adolescent, and adult patients. I also led diabetes and weight management classes. All of this occurred under supervision of the preceptor.

Community:

1. SuperKids Nutrition (online rotation). In this rotation, I mainly participated in the development of handouts, recipes, and social media messages for diverse platforms, and assisted in the development of the newest website for this rotation. The main goal was to make nutrition education accessible, easy to understand, and applicable in everyday life.
2. Viva Nutrition at Briggs' Family Pediatrics. In this rotation, I shadowed and eventually provided one-on-one nutritional counseling to a variety of pediatric, adolescent, and adult patients, both in English and Spanish. I also developed multiple nutrition education handouts for patients in both languages.
3. Heritage Health and Housing–Food and Nutrition Services. In this rotation, I completed nutrition assessments and provided nutritional counseling one-on-one, group education, and food demonstrations to HIV/AIDS participants. I also assisted in the food pantry and congregate meals that were offered on a daily basis to the participants.

Foodservice:

1. The Calhoun School. I was involved in food preparation, lunches, and catering serving for 650 or more people daily. I reviewed menus, assessed meal service, and conducted workshops to chefs on food safety and food allergens.

For the elective rotations, I spent 4 additional weeks at Mary Manning Walsh Nursing Home and Heritage Health and Housing–Food and Nutrition Services.

How have you been involved professionally?
I am currently a member of the Pediatric Nutrition and Nutrition Education for the Public Dietetic Practice Groups. I try to attend conferences related to my work (e.g., Pediatric and Adult Weight Management) to keep current with the literature and network with fellow colleagues.

What honors or awards have you received?
I was on the Dean's List all 4 years of undergraduate classes and graduated summa cum laude from Queens College. I was on the Presidential Honor Roll my freshman year, and I have been a member of the Golden Key International Honor Society since September 2007.

Briefly describe your career path in dietetics. What are you doing now?
After completing the Dietetic Internship program and for the past 2 years, I have been working full time as a Registered Dietitian Nutritionist at a community health center in the South Bronx in New York, called Urban Health Plan, Inc., where I do nutrition counseling for a variety of populations both in English and Spanish: in pediatrics, providing nutrition counseling to families with newborns, toddlers, and school-age children; in obstetrics, assisting prenatal and postpartum women with healthy eating and weight gain throughout the pregnancy and after they give birth; and in adult patients, providing nutrition counseling for various conditions such as underweight, overweight, obesity, appetite issues, diabetes, hyperlipidemia, hypertension, HIV, etc. I am also actively involved in the preparation and execution of multiple nutrition outreach activities promoting nutrition education, healthy eating and lifestyle, and disease prevention and management for clinic patients and the community at large.

For the past 2.5 years, I have also been working as an Adjunct Lecturer at Queens College, City University of New York, where I teach two undergraduate courses in the

Nutrition and Exercise Sciences program. One of the courses I teach—Nutrition for the Exercise Professionals—addresses the foundation of nutrition assessment and intervention across the life cycle and for diseases commonly encountered by the exercise professional. The other course I teach—Internship in Exercise Sciences—is an in-depth, structured, practical experience in a formalized program dealing with fitness and health enhancement of individuals. This opportunity to teach came to me as I graduated with my master's degree in 2013 and after 4 years of working as a teaching assistant in the Family, Nutrition, and Exercise Sciences department at Queens College.

What excites you about dietetics and the future of our profession?

What excites me the most is that it is becoming more mainstream to have an interdisciplinary approach to health and disease prevention and management; medical providers are working along dietitians to offer the best care to patients, promoting lifestyle modifications to help reduce the risk of developing chronic diseases and obesity. In addition, I am very excited about the continued growing opportunities available to us in this field.

How is teamwork important to you in your position? How have you been involved in team projects?

Teamwork is vital! I work on team projects constantly, whenever I am involved in outreach activities, expos, and presentations. I enjoy being a part of the team, assisting with the creative, organizational, and/or logistics aspects and, at times, also assuming a leadership role. I am currently involved in an interdisciplinary, integrative Life Enhancement Program for teens and their families, which is expected to begin this year, that would promote healthy lifestyle for the family as a whole.

What words of wisdom do you have for future dietetics professionals?

It may take time or you may know right away, but find a path that excites you and that you are passionate about. Enjoying what you do and looking forward to going to work every day makes life much better and much less stressful. Further your education by taking continuing education classes; attending seminars, workshops, or conferences; or auditing a class; this will help you stay current with your knowledge since nutrition is a science that keeps evolving!

References

1. Cassell J. *Carry the Flame: The History of the American Dietetic Association.* Chicago: The American Dietetic Association; 1990.
2. Otis FA. A combination theory and practice course for student dietitians. *J Am Diet Assoc.* 1925;3:138–140.
3. Section on Education of the American Dietetic Association. Standardization of courses for student dietitians in hospitals. *J Am Diet Assoc.* 1926;12:171–176.
4. Northrop MW. The training of student dietitians. *J Am Diet Assoc.* 1929;5:208–211.
5. Professional Education Section. Chairman's Summary. *J Am Diet Assoc.* 1940;16: 1016–1018.
6. Accreditation Council for Education in Nutrition and Dietetics. 2012 Standards for Technician Education Programs; Dietitian Education Programs; Didactic Programs in Nutrition and Dietetics; Internship Programs in Nutrition and Dietetics; Foreign Dietitian Education Programs; International Dietitian Education Programs. Available at: http://www.eatrightacend.org/ACEND/. Accessed January 11, 2016.
7. Academy of Nutrition and Dietetics. ACEND Mission. Available at: http://www.eatrightacend.org/ACEND/content.aspx?id=6442485282. Accessed January 11, 2016.

8. Academy of Nutrition and Dietetics. ACEND Board Members. Available at: http://www .eatrightacend.org/ACEND/content.aspx?id=6442485267. Accessed January 11, 2016.

9. Academy of Nutrition and Dietetics. ACEND Peer Program Reviewers. Available at: http://www.eatrightacend.org/ACEND/content.aspx?id=6442485283. Accessed January 11, 2016.

10. Academy of Nutrition and Dietetics. Procedure for Complaints Against Accredited Programs. Available at: http://www.eatright.org/ACEND/content.aspx?id=7975. Accessed May 5, 2012.

11. Academy of Nutrition and Dietetics. What Is a Registered Dietitian? Available at: http:// www.eatright.org/BecomeanRDorDTR/content.aspx?id=8142. Accessed March 20, 2016.

12. Academy of Nutrition and Dietetics. What Is a Dietetic Technician, Registered? Available at: http://www.eatright.org/BecomeanRDorDTR/content.aspx?id=8142. Accessed March 20, 2016.

13. Academy of Nutrition and Dietetics. The Basics for Students. Available at: http://www .eatrightpro.org/resource/career/become-an-rdn-or-dtr/high-school-students/the-basics . Accessed January 11, 2016.

14. Academy of Nutrition and Dietetics. Accredited Education Programs. Available at: http:// www.eatrightacend.org/ACEND/content.aspx?id=6442485414. Accessed January 10, 2016.

15. Moore M, Kearsley G. *Distance Education: A Systems View.* Belmont, CA: Wadsworth; 1996:2.

16. Hansen RS. Distance learning pros and cons. Available at: http://www.quintcareers.com /distance_learning_pros-cons.html. Accessed March 20, 2016.

17. Seifer S, Connors K. Improved student learning and community health: the CCPH faculty service learning institute. *Acad Med.* 2000;75:533–534.

18. Chabot JM, Holben DH. Integrating service-learning into dietetics and nutrition education. *Topics Clin Nutr.* 2003;18(3):177–184.

19. Williams AG, Hall KJ, Shadix K, Stokes DM. *Creating Your Career Portfolio: At-a-Glance Guide for Dietitians.* Upper Saddle River, NJ: Prentice-Hall; 2005.

20. Academy of Nutrition and Dietetics. 2015 Compensation & Benefits Survey of the Dietetics Profession. Available at: http://www.eatrightstore.org/product/B2112E17-FF41-418C-8208-27539D3E5C0F. May 6, 2016.

21. Academy of Nutrition and Dietetics. Advanced Degrees. Available at: http://www .eatrightpro.org/resources/career/professional-development/advanced-degrees. Accessed January 9, 2016.

22. Academy of Nutrition and Dietetics. Accredited Dietetic Education Programs. Available at: http://www.eatrightacend.org/ACEND/content.aspx?id=6442485414. Accessed January 9, 2016.

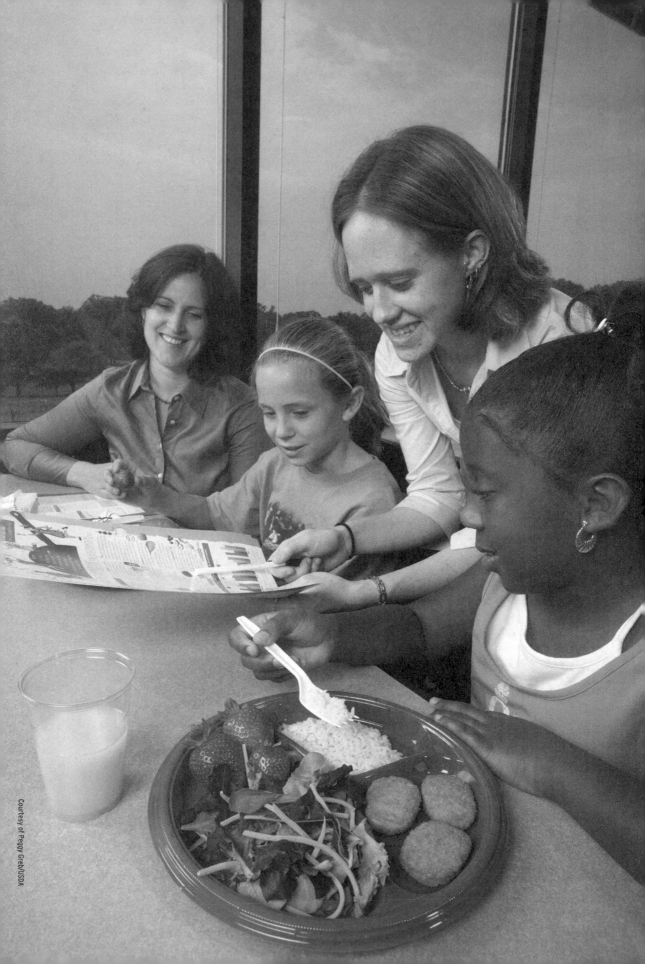

The Supervised Practice Experience

Trying Your Wings

For students wishing to become credentialed dietetics professionals, nothing is more nerve-wracking or more exciting than the process of applying for and being admitted to the supervised practice experience. Students in Nutrition and Dietetics Technician Programs participate in a 450-hour supervised practice experience; those pursuing the Registered Dietitian Nutritionist (RDN) credential must successfully complete at least 1,200 hours. This chapter discusses the supervised practice experience and how one prepares for, applies for, and gets the most out of this critical step on the path to the dietetics profession.

Supervised practice is the critical time when you have the opportunity to try out the application of theory in the "real world." It is the time when you really see what dietetics professionals do in a variety of work settings, how they spend their time, the decisions they make, the challenges they face, the joys and trials of the job, and the "politics" of the workplace. The dietetics professionals who act as preceptors will become some of the most instrumental people in your professional development. Most of these individuals are not paid to work with students or interns; they do it out of the goodness of their hearts and their desire to help the next generation of food and nutrition professionals. In other words, they are often the "unsung heroes" in the story of dietetics education and training. Whether your supervised practice takes place in one facility or in multiple sites, an incredible amount of planning and coordination has taken place "behind the scenes" to make this learning experience the best possible.

Competencies for the Supervised Practice Component

Just as the Accreditation Council for Education in Nutrition and Dietetics (ACEND) has outlined specific "Core Knowledge" for the academic part of your dietetics education, there are also specific "Core Competencies" for the supervised practice component of both nutrition and dietetics technician and dietitian education programs.[1,2] As you read through the "Core Competencies," you will see that performance-based and action verbs are used to demonstrate that these are hands-on skills to be developed, readying you for practice in the real world.

Just as with the didactic portion of dietetics education, the supervised practice competencies have been developed from practice audits and research with practicing dietetics professionals who understand what an entry-level professional should be able to do when arriving on his or her first job. The supervised practice experience is exactly what the name implies. It is a time when you, as a student or intern, can "practice" the competencies expected of a professional while under "supervision." You can hone your skills and get a feel for what the day-to-day activities are like for a dietitian or nutrition and dietetics technician in a relatively low-risk environment.

Although ACEND dictates that a minimum number of hours must be included in supervised practice, the division of these hours among the different competencies to be achieved is not mandated. Each dietetics program looks at its goals, desired outcomes, and resources and decides how to divide the hours. In other words, to meet the 450- or 1,200-hour requirement, the program does not have to provide one-third of the hours in community nutrition, one-third in foodservice management, and one-third in clinical nutrition. As long as the program can demonstrate by outcome assessment that its graduates are meeting the core competencies, the faculty can design the program to take the best advantage of its resources and meet the specific needs of its constituencies.

When Does Supervised Practice Occur?

Supervised practice programs for nutrition and dietetics technicians must be a minimum of 450 hours. Supervised practice programs for dietitians must be a minimum of 1,200 hours. The program may opt to include more hours of training if needed to achieve the program goals. This training occurs at different points, depending on the type of program in which the student is enrolled. Some students graduate from a Didactic Program in Dietetics (DPD) and then are admitted to a post-baccalaureate Dietetic Internship (DI). DIs vary in length. Some are as brief and intense as 6 months, during which interns work 50 hours per week to complete the requirements. Others may last 1 or 2 years, especially if graduate coursework or a master's degree is combined with the supervised practice program.

Students in Coordinated Programs in Dietetics (CPs) are involved in supervised practice concurrently with their didactic coursework. Some programs may start the supervised practice experience during the junior year and extend the acquisition of the 1,200 hours over three or four semesters. The Academy of Nutrition and Dietetics website also lists 23 CPs that provide the opportunity for students to combined graduate coursework with supervised practice, culminating in a master's degree.[3] Likewise, Nutrition and Dietetics Technician Programs also have the 450 hours of supervised practice interspersed and sequenced with the didactic coursework.

The Dietetic Internship Shortage

It is common knowledge that the number of students seeking admission to dietetic internships is far greater than the number of available internships. The ACEND website on www.eatright.org provides a table showing the percent change in number of openings, applicants, and applicants matched to DI programs participating in the computer matching process since 1993. The latest figures from 2015 show that only 49% of the students who applied for an internship were actually matched to one. The 2015 data indicate that there were 3,158 internship openings for 5,853 applicants.[4]

Why is this shortage occurring? The answer is a complex one. Interest in food and nutrition among the public has skyrocketed, and more and more individuals are interested in pursuing a career in a food/nutrition-related profession. Because RDNs are touted as "the nutrition experts," it is logical that students flock to dietetic education programs. Growing program enrollment in higher education institutions is viewed positively by administrators.

At the same time, increases in healthcare costs and legislative efforts to control these costs in healthcare systems, such as the Patient Protection and Affordable Care Act, have caused sweeping changes. Since most dietetic internships are located in/sponsored by hospitals, cost reduction efforts and ever-increasing bureaucracy have made many chief executive officers and other hospital administrators leery of adding new programs. Heightened focus on liability issues and patient privacy add to the concerns. Many internships are forced to be solely self-supporting, and thus, students must be charged ever-increasing tuition/fees to cover their costs. Finding facilities willing to take dietetic students/interns is increasingly challenging because typically facilities and preceptors are not paid to participate in dietetic education. Thus, the work of planning experiences as well as directing and evaluating students is an additional demand on RDNs who may already be overworked and underpaid. The bottom line is that starting up a new internship is a tough business!

Making the Decision: Coordinated Program versus Dietetic Internship

The above saga and statistics should make aspiring students think deeply about which type of supervised practice program would be best for them. Many people view applying to and being admitted to a CP in Dietetics as the logical alternative to the scarce dietetic internship placement scenario. However, one must remember that as more students decide to opt for CP application, this makes that route increasingly competitive as well.

Currently, there are 56 CPs in Dietetics and 246 DIs in the United States.[3] As previously discussed, CPs combine the supervised practice experience with the academic degree program. These programs were initially designed to speed up the preparation of dietitians by combining the hands-on experience with the degree program and eliminating the post-baccalaureate internship requirement. This means that students in these programs could conceivably be RDN-eligible in a shorter period of time. However, as the list of ACEND competencies becomes longer, programs may increase in length as well. Students, desiring to make themselves more competitive, may opt to earn secondary majors or minors to enhance their transcript. This phenomenon may also increase the length of a student's educational program. Many supervised practice programs also expect to see dietetics-related or other work experience on the student's application. Such work experience may be pursued in the summer months, thus sometimes reducing the opportunity of taking summer classes to hasten graduation. The idea that the bachelor of science (BS) degree is a "4-year degree" is rapidly falling by the wayside as more and more students take 5 years or longer to complete a baccalaureate program in nutrition or dietetics, plus a secondary major or minor(s) and pertinent work experience.

As with any decision, there are pros and cons to be considered. Students should consider numerous factors before deciding which route to take. Just living close to a particular program doesn't mean that it is the best program for you. Programs have strengths and weaknesses, advantages and limitations, and a culture or "personality"—just like individuals. Wise students do their homework ahead of time by visiting program websites; actually visiting the program to talk to faculty and students, if possible; and checking out program statistics before making the all-important decision to apply for admission.

CPs often draw their students from a more regional area, whereas DIs may attract students from across the country. Because supervised practice hours are built into the degree program, CPs are intense and allow for few unrestricted electives. However, CP graduates are immediately eligible to sit for the RDN exam, and thus enter practice sooner than their internship-bound classmates. Students who decide to enroll in a didactic program followed by an internship may have more unrestricted electives; thus, it may be easier for them to gain a minor or second major during their undergraduate program. Interns may be able to combine graduate coursework or a full master's degree program along with their internship. As mentioned earlier, there are also some master's-level CPs. Twenty-six of the 56 CPs culminate in a graduate degree. Obviously, each type of program has its pros and cons, and only you can decide which type of program is best for you.

Another great resource for decision making is the *Applicant Guide to Supervised Practice*, a publication of Nutrition and Dietetic Educators and Preceptors (NDEP), an organizational unit in the Academy. This publication is updated annually and may be purchased from the online store at www.eatright.org.[5] Your program director also may have a copy on reserve in his or her office, in your school library, or posted online in the dietetics program information. Not all supervised practice programs may choose to include their information in this publication. However, the document contains a wealth of information about supervised practice programs that choose to submit information. Information includes the cost of the program, entrance requirements, factors considered in evaluating applications, kinds of facilities used for experiences, typical numbers of students applying, acceptance rates, and other information that is difficult to find from traditional resources.

Every year, many DIs host open houses so that prospective applicants can learn more about the various programs available. Keep in touch with your didactic program director, because he or she may be notified about these open houses. Also, during the annual Food and Nutrition Conference and Exhibition (FNCE) of the Academy, DIs often set up displays and information tables about their programs at the Student Reception.

A good way to acquire information about supervised practice is to visit the Student Center website, an area on the public Academy website (www .eatright.org) that is chock-full of great information for students. The Members Only section of the Academy website offers additional information for Academy student members about improving one's chances of getting an internship placement, student tips for success in supervised practice, and information about the availability of DIs.[6]

Other sources for information and guidance about the DI application process are the websites set up by DIs themselves. Because being selected for a DI is increasingly competitive, students can benefit from these informative sites and gain insight into what each program may be looking for in applicants.

Distance Internships

A relatively new phenomenon in the world of supervised practice is the "distance internship." As distance education didactic programs in dietetics have grown, the idea of distance internships has also become a reality. The Academy website currently lists 19 internships that offer distance education options.[7] To gain admission to these kinds of programs, a student must obtain the application guidelines from the internship and then work on their own to set up sites to obtain supervised practice experiences prior to applying for program admission. Typically the applicant must present to the distance internship program a complete listing of facilities and preceptors in their geographic area who have agreed to work with the student as part of their application packet. Every program has its own policies and procedures. If this sort of program sounds as if it may meet your needs, visit the websites of these programs and see whether such a program may be right for you.

Setting up all the sites and finding preceptors can be an incredibly challenging and time-consuming experience, so give yourself plenty of time to work toward this goal in order to meet application deadlines. Hospital-based clinical sites are often the most difficult to orchestrate. Networking with local dietitians while you are a student can sometimes help smooth the path later on if you plan to try to put together your own distance internship program. Conducting "cold calls" to ask whether a facility or RDN would be willing to work with you is very difficult if the student is unknown to the facility, so building relationships early is highly recommended! Join your local district dietetic association as a student. Be an Academy of Nutrition and Dietetics student member, which automatically makes you a member of your state dietetic association. Attend the professional meetings of these organizations and get your name and face known. Volunteer your time to help local RDNs with projects. All of these activities can pay big dividends in the long run when you are trying to set up sites and find preceptors!

Individualized Supervised Practice Pathways (ISPPs)

Individualized supervised practice pathways, or ISPPs, were introduced in September 2011 by the Academy. These programs provide students the opportunity to gain the required knowledge and skills for dietetics practice by working under the guidance of individual practitioners with direction from an ACEND-accredited dietetics program. Individuals who can take advantage of an ISPP are limited to the following:

- Pathway 1: Didactic Program in Dietetics (DPD) program graduates who hold a DPD Verification Statement and have a baccalaureate degree granted by a U.S. regionally accredited college/university. Before a DPD graduate can apply to an ISPP, they first must have applied to a dietetic internship but did NOT match in the computer matching process.
- Pathway 2: Doctoral program graduates. For these individuals, a DPD Verification Statement is not required. The doctoral degree must be granted by a U.S. regionally accredited college/university. Check the ISPP site on the ACEND website (http://www.eatrightacend .org/ACEND/content.aspx?id=6442485529) for more detailed information.[8]

Applying for the Supervised Practice Experience

The supervised practice experience application process can be broken down into the following steps.

Step 1: Gain Dietetics-Related Work Experience

Start early by gaining dietetics-related work experience. This may be paid experience or volunteer experience. Gain experience in as many different areas of dietetics practice as you can. You will learn much about the breadth and depth of the profession of dietetics, which will better prepare you to take advantage of your supervised practice experiences. Some supervised practice programs may require you to have a certain number of hours of work experience before you apply to the program. Such work experience is highly recommended for all students and will only strengthen your application. You can obtain dietetics-related work experience in a number of ways:

- Volunteer with a Women, Infants, and Children (WIC) program.
- Deliver Meals-on-Wheels to the elderly.
- Work at a health fair with a dietetics professional.
- Work as a diet aide in a hospital or long-term care facility.
- Shadow dietitians in various areas of dietetics practice, and observe what they do and how they do it.

- Gain work experience in foodservice operations in food preparation and service. Look for part-time jobs in hospital or nursing home kitchens, restaurants, summer camps, or other foodservice operations. While waitstaff experience is good to have, back-of-the-house food preparation experience is invaluable.
- Look for shadowing or volunteer opportunities with dietetics professionals who work in nontraditional areas of practice, such as those working with the media or on the Internet; RDNs in private practice counseling, consulting, sales, and marketing; and other entrepreneurs.

Step 2: Investigate the Available Supervised Practice Programs

Investigate the wide array of available supervised practice programs. The Academy website (www.eatright.org) has a complete list of CPs, DIs, and Nutrition and Dietetics Technician Programs; this includes a brief description of the program, the program director's name, the website for the program, and contact information for the program director.[9,10]

Visit the websites of the various programs, and, if you need further information, contact the program director. Take advantage of any open house opportunities that the program may provide or call and ask if you can make special arrangements to visit the program. Read the program description carefully to determine whether the focus of the program is in line with your interests.

Step 3: Narrow Your Choices

Narrow your choices and decide on the programs to which you wish to apply. Remember that putting together a "letter-perfect" application takes considerable time and effort, so be selective in your efforts. Also, do not "put all your eggs in one basket." Applying to only one program can be risky, because competition is strong for supervised practice placements. Applying to only one program and not being selected can be a devastating experience. Carefully think through your top five to eight choices. Think long term. Do not pick a supervised practice program because it is convenient or because it has a stipend or because a close friend is applying there as well. Keep your long-term goals in mind and strategize on how you can best achieve them.

Step 4: Become Familiar with the Dietetic Internship Centralized Application System (DICAS)

Most dietetic internships now use the Dietetic Internship Centralized Application System, or DICAS, for handling internship applications. Applications are submitted through DICAS between specific dates and times for each internship appointment period. See the ACEND website, Computer Matching Policy and Procedures section, for further information on DICAS.[11] Coordinated dietetics programs do not participate in DICAS or in computer matching.

Step 5: Register for Computer Matching

Computer matching is the process by which internship placement decisions are made. The computer matching for dietetic internships is handled by

D&D Digital (http://www.dnddigital.com/).[12] Whereas CPs and Nutrition and Dietetics Technician Programs have their own applicant selection processes, students who are applying for post-baccalaureate DIs participate in national computer matching for internship placement. A few internships do not participate in computer matching because they accept only graduates of their sponsoring institution. (For example, a university-sponsored internship accepts applications only from graduates of that university's DPD program.) Otherwise, all other internships must participate in the computer-matching process.

Computer matching is a contractual agreement between the Academy and D&D Digital Systems, whereby you are matched through a computerized process with the highest-ranked program that offers you a position. Computer matching uses the prioritized list of programs to which you applied and the internship's prioritized list of their applicants to make the matches. There is a $50 charge to applicants to participate in this process.

Much thought should be given to prioritizing the programs to which you have applied. You must remember that your highest priority match is the one you must accept, so this step is a very important one. You register and prioritize your internship choices online at the D&D Digital website. Once you have prioritized your applications, be sure to keep a copy for your records. Your priority listing may be changed even after you have submitted it, up to a specific date during the application process. Check with D&D Digital about the final date changes can be made.

Step 6: Seek Letters of Reference/Recommendations

Pay attention to the program's requirements for letters of reference or recommendations. Also be aware of the Family Educational Rights and Privacy Act (FERPA), which requires that you give permission for a faculty member to release information about you, such as your grade point average (GPA), class rank, and other specific information that is not part of your public records.[13] Check with your university about how they are ensuring that FERPA requirements are being followed.

Be professional in your approach when asking individuals to write references or recommendations for you. Do not wait until the last minute! Many didactic program directors and other faculty members are inundated with requests for letters and recommendations by students who are all applying to supervised practice programs at the same time. It is critical that you provide as much information as possible to this person so that he or she can write an accurate and insightful recommendation for you. One idea might be to provide the recommendation writer with a copy of your application to the program. At minimum, you should provide a current résumé and a copy of your personal statement. Give a specific date by which you need to have the recommendations completed, allowing a little extra time so that if the individual falls behind in the task, you won't be late in meeting the application deadline.

As part of your DICAS application procedure, you will be asked to provide the names and email addresses of individuals providing references for you. These individuals will be sent an email with instructions on how to submit their recommendations for you online through the DICAS process.

Step 7: Send Official Transcripts of All Academic Coursework

Official transcripts of your academic coursework from all colleges and universities you have attended must be submitted as part of the DICAS process. "Official" transcripts are in sealed envelopes, are stamped with the seal of the university, and are typically mailed directly from the university registrar's office to the address you designate. If you attended multiple schools, remember that you must obtain transcripts from all schools, and you must allow time for this process. Remember that "Degree Granted" needs to be stamped on the transcript from schools where you received your degree(s). Official copies of transcripts are mailed to the DICAS Transcript Department, P.O. Box 9118, Watertown, MA 02472, to become part of your centralized application.

Step 8: Proofread Your Application

Have your dietetics program director and/or academic advisor proofread a draft of your application. Remember that your application may be the only representation the internship will have of you. Grammatical mistakes and typographical errors may make the difference in whether your application is rated lower than someone else's. The smallest things can make a huge difference in your success.

Step 9: Make a Copy of Your Application

Make a copy of your application for your files. It is always important for you to keep a copy of such important documents in case of computer system malfunction or some other unforeseen circumstance.

Step 10: Check the Due Date

Check the date when the applications are due. Typically, this date is in mid-February for a fall supervised practice start date or mid-September for a January start date. If you are applying to a graduate program as well as to the supervised practice program, check the deadlines for this application, because the dates may be different. Be sure to see if you must be admitted to their graduate school first before you can apply to the internship.

The Interview as Part of the Admission Process

Some supervised practice programs may include an interview as part of the admission process. Often this is a telephone interview. Prepare for this interview as you would for a job interview. Check the date and time for the interview and be punctual. This is especially important if you are located in a different time zone than the internship program. It's all too easy to confuse times and accidentally miss a call! Before the interview, make a list of questions you would like to ask, and think through questions that might be posed to you. Take the call in a quiet location where you will not be interrupted. Also, consider taking the call on a "landline phone" rather than on a cell phone, where you might lose the signal or otherwise get disconnected. Remember to smile while you are talking. It shows in your voice! Be enthusiastic and upbeat. Even though the interview committee can't see you, they will be able to sense the energy and excitement in your voice. Some internships may opt for a video conference rather than audio only. If this is the case, be sure to dress professionally and conduct your call in a neat and uncluttered location.

Match Day for Dietetic Internship Placement

The day on which you find out if you have matched for an internship placement is one filled with anticipation and excitement. The dates for "Match Day" are announced by the Academy and D&D Digital Systems each year. Your DPD director can provide this information for you. Students who apply for a DI starting in the fall are notified of the match results on a specific "Notification Day" in April. Students applying for a DI starting in the spring are notified on a "Notification Day" in November.

Before the notification date arrives, you will be sent specific login information and a password so that you can access the D&D Digital website at the specified date and time to see the results of the computer-matching process.

What happens if you do not receive a match? It's not the end of the world. Sometimes programs do not fill all their available internship slots. D&D Digital will post on its website a list of programs that have open spaces and want those openings advertised. This is known as the "second round match." If you give permission, your name and contact information will be sent to these internships and to your DPD director. Your DPD director can work with you to look at the internships that have open positions and evaluate whether you'd like to submit your application to one of those programs. Each year, many students who did not receive a match in the computer process eventually receive an internship placement in this "secondary" process. Or, you may elect to wait until the next round of computer matching and reapply.

Once you have finished your academic program, your DPD director will provide you with a Verification Statement indicating that you have completed your final DPD coursework. Your DPD director must sign this form, and you must send it to your internship director before starting the supervised practice experience. Pack your bags! You're on your way!

Being Successful in the Supervised Practice Experience

Whether you are participating in a DI, a CP, or a Nutrition and Dietetics Technician Program, the supervised practice experience is one of the most exciting times in your professional preparation. It is vital that you take advantage of every learning opportunity during this critical time. The following are some things to keep in mind during your supervised practice experience:

- Establish a cordial and cooperative relationship with your preceptor(s) and share your interests and professional goals. Look at this internship experience as if you were beginning a new job. Always look and act professionally as a member of the organization's team. Remember that you are still learning. Confidence is a good thing, but do not act like you know all the answers!
- Come to your experience prepared to take advantage of this wonderful opportunity you've been given. Do your "homework" before each learning experience by reviewing your notes and looking over readings that relate to that rotation. Before you begin each day, formulate

objectives and think through what you want to accomplish. At the end of the day, do a quick assessment of how successful you were in reaching your goals, and reformulate new goals for the following day.

- Remember "the big picture" and use systems thinking. Do not get so engrossed in one activity that you miss what else is going on around you. Analyze what you are doing and how it relates to everything else in your unit, department, or the organization as a whole. Every decision or action has repercussions throughout the organization. Take time to make those connections and learn from them.
- Plan your time wisely and accomplish as much as you can. If you are in the middle of an important task with which you have been charged, finish the task. Others may be depending on your completion of that assignment. Remember that professionals often are salaried, not hourly, employees. Stay until the job is done and your responsibilities have been fulfilled. Do not be a "clock watcher"!
- Be flexible, positive, enthusiastic, and polite. Demonstrate initiative, but remember there are limits to your authority. If you're not sure what those boundaries are, check with your preceptor. And finally, treat others the way you'd want to be treated. Remember that the professionals you work within your supervised practice experience may be references for you for future employment or other opportunities. Do not burn any bridges!

When Supervised Practice Is Completed

Completion of your supervised practice experience signifies the end of the second step in the three-step process of becoming a credentialed dietetics professional. If you are a CP or Nutrition and Dietetics Technician Program student, one Verification Statement will be issued to you, showing that you have completed both the academic and supervised practice requirements to sit for the national credentialing exam. CP students are eligible to take the national Registration Examination for Dietitian Nutritionists, whereas Nutrition and Dietetics Technician graduates are eligible for the national Registration Examination for Nutrition and Dietetics Technicians.

For individuals completing a DI, a second Verification Statement will be provided showing that the intern has met the supervised practice requirements. This statement will be added to the academic Verification Statement from the DPD program, thus indicating that all requirements are met and that the individual is ready to move to step 3, sitting for the national Registration Examination for Dietitian Nutritionists.

Supervised practice provides the required hands-on work experience for you to be ready for the national credentialing examination as a dietetics professional. It is a time of hard work and learning, networking and growth, excitement and promise. The people you meet and work with during this time are vital mentors for your professional growth. Take advantage of gaining everything you can from the experience, and when you are a dietetics professional, perhaps you'll have the opportunity to guide the supervised practice experience for another aspiring professional!

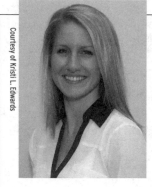

Profile of a Professional

Kristi L. Edwards, MS, RDN, LDN, CLC

Clinical Dietitian
Regional One Health, Memphis, Tennessee

Education:
BS in Dietetics, University of Tennessee at Martin, Martin, Tennessee
MS in Clinical Nutrition, University of Memphis, Memphis, Tennessee

How did you first hear about dietetics and decide to become a Registered Dietitian?

Growing up, I was involved in sports and competitive gymnastics and cheerleading (I can still do a standing back tuck!). I quickly learned that good nutrition resulted in better performance and improved energy. As I grew older, I recognized my passion for helping and teaching others. I knew I wanted to do something in the medical field, and my favorite class was Anatomy and Physiology. When I learned of a career that combined my love for nutrition and desire to help others improve their health, I knew dietetics was the perfect fit.

What was your route to registration?

I graduated summa cum laude from the University of Tennessee at Martin, where I obtained a bachelor's degree in Dietetics and a minor in Business Administration. I received the Outstanding Dietetics Student Award of my class. I then went on to complete the combined dietetic internship and master's program at the University of Memphis, where I had the privilege of spending 10 months with a Registered Dietitian in the bone marrow transplant clinic at St. Jude Children's Research Hospital. This was an unparalleled experience. The internship also included rotating through hospitals, clinics, gyms, and culinary institutions in Memphis and the surrounding area.

Where did you complete your supervised practice experience?

The director of the didactic program at the University of Tennessee at Martin communicated with hospitals in the surrounding area to provide myself and other dietetics students with valuable field experience. I also completed over 1,200 hours of supervised practice experience in my completion of the combined internship and master's program at the University of Memphis.

How are you involved professionally?

I am a member of the Academy of Nutrition and Dietetics as well as the Memphis Academy of Nutrition and Dietetics (MAND). I've contributed nutrition blogs to the MAND website previously, and I plan to soon run for an officer position. I am also a member of the Memphis Area Lactation Consultant Association. During my time at the University of Memphis, I obtained my Certified Lactation Counselor (CLC) credential.

What honors or awards have you received?

While obtaining my undergraduate degree in Dietetics at the University of Tennessee at Martin, I was invited to join Rho Lambda, Gamma Beta Phi, and Phi Eta Sigma National Honor Societies. I also received Outstanding Dietetics Student Award of my senior class at the University of Tennessee at Martin.

Briefly describe your career path in dietetics. What are you doing now?

Looking back on my time as an intern and student, I was open to many different possibilities in the field of dietetics. I loved my time as a graduate assistant at St. Jude Children's Research Hospital, where I learned a great deal about nutrition in pediatrics and lactation. My other interests as an intern included diabetes, chronic kidney disease, and corporate wellness.

I am currently a clinical dietitian with Regional One Health in Memphis, and I am able to apply knowledge gained from each of the aforementioned areas of interest to my daily responsibilities. We do have the occasional pediatric patient. Knowledge of nutrition and lactation is applied to mothers on the maternity floors, and chronic kidney disease patients and diabetes patients are seen and educated daily. As I continue to gain experience in the burn, trauma, high-risk obstetrics, intensive care, rehabilitation, and long-term acute care units at Regional One Health, I am convinced that this has been (and continues to be) an opportunity beyond compare. I learn so many new things each and every day, and I value the teamwork and the trust of the physicians with whom I work.

I also write bimonthly nutrition articles for *At Home Memphis and Mid South* magazine as well as volunteer with GROW Memphis and Junior League of Memphis.

What excites you about dietetics and the future of our profession?
Knowledge of nutrition and its impact on health is growing. It is predicted that employment of dietitians will increase 20% from 2010 and 2020, according to the U.S. Bureau of Labor Statistics. This is faster than the average growth of all other occupations. As we continue to practice evidenced-based medical nutrition therapy, individuals and organizations continue to see the impact of our services. As we continue to perform research, doctors continue to gain our trust in the clinical setting. Rates of reimbursement for our services continue to increase. I have high hopes for the future of the dietetics profession.

How is teamwork important to you in your position? How have you been involved in team projects?
Teamwork is at the top of the list in terms of most important things a multidisciplinary approach requires in the clinical setting. I am a big fan of the sharing of information. At Regional One Health, dietitians educate anyone and everyone from patients to foodservice workers to doctors and managers. We are constantly updating our standards of practice to reflect up-to-date evidence-based nutrition information.

What words of wisdom do you have for future dietetics professionals?
Never let someone tell you that you cannot do something. You can do anything if you put your mind to it. I am a quotes person, and one of my favorites is, "First they'll ask you why you're doing it . . . then they'll ask you how you did it." Work hard, and be open to the opportunities that present themselves.

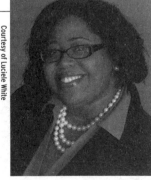

Courtesy of Luciele White

Profile of a Professional

Luciele White, RD

Regional Customer Experience Manager
Touchpoint Support Services, Austin, Texas

Education:
Bachelor's in Baking and Pastry Arts, Culinary Nutrition, Johnson and Wales University, Providence, Rhode Island

How did you first hear about dietetics and decide to become a Registered Dietitian?
Well, I first heard about nutrition while I was in high school, but I got serious when I was at Johnson and Wales University when they decided to offer a new major "Culinary Nutrition." When I found out that I could have an impact on what people ate and how to help to heal with food, I was all in!

What was your route to registration (internship, coordinated program, preplanned experience, etc.)?

I had a very traditional route to registration. I got matched to my internship through the computer-matching process.

At what college or university did you receive your entry-level education?

I received my undergraduate degree from Johnson and Wales University in Providence, Rhode Island. I received two bachelor's degrees, one in Baking and Pastry Arts and the second in Culinary Nutrition.

Where did you complete your supervised practice experience?

I completed my supervised practice at the University of Virginia Health Systems in Charlottesville, Virginia.

How are you involved professionally?

I am an active member of:

- The Academy of Nutrition and Dietetics
- The Culinary Professionals DPG
- The Beryl Institute
- The Association of Training and Development

Briefly describe your career path in dietetics. What are you doing now?

I took a very untraditional route to dietetics. I started out on the culinary side of things. I went to culinary school and started out pursuing pastries and desserts. Then I was given the opportunity to combine my passion for food with my passion for helping people. I received a scholarship from Morrison Management Specialist/Compass Group USA, which not only allowed me to cover my internship tuition in its totality, but also provided me with a job opportunity after graduation. So I have had the privilege of growth and exposure for the past 12 years. I started working as a clinical unit RD and then transitioned into a foodservice operational role as a Production Manager, really working as an Executive Chef. Then I moved into an Assistant Director role for the Food and Nutrition Department where I was able to help with my community initiatives for heart health, diabetes, and pediatric wellness programs. I was eager to get back to University of Virginia, and a position became available to work in their Patient Services department of Food and Nutrition Service (FNS), so I came back and had the chance to help improve the patient services menus and relationships between the clinical teams and the support teams of FNS.

Presently I am working as a Customer Experience Manager, where I create a positive experience for our patients, associates, clients, and internal team members, helping to develop and empower people with the tools and skills to foster a positive first and lasting impression. I help to monitor and track outcomes and train others in how to better communicate caring and compassion to our patients. It's a far cry from just thinking of how a nutritionally adequate meal can help to heal a person. Now I have the ability to affect the way that caretakers (associates), leaders, and future leaders will care for our patients and their families.

What excites you about dietetics and the future of our profession?

What excites me about dietetics is that it is something that affects everyone regardless of nationality, religion, race, or creed! We have the ability to help all people participate in a healthy life just by teaching and sharing our knowledge of how food and nutrients affect the body. Food is as universal as music or love. All cultures use food as a form of celebration, to express creativity, and to provide a sense of comfort and nostalgia, but they also all relate to food as a source of healing! The future of our profession is exciting because it has grown and continues to grow past the traditional boundaries of just a healthcare/clinical setting. Our input as RDs is being infused into all facets of our everyday life of health and wellness, we are more visible as the experts that we are in the media (television, radio, social media, blogs, etc.), we are in supermarkets, and we are in space (NASA), research, sports, business product development, prevention, etc. The possibilities are endless!

How is teamwork important to you in your position? How have you been involved in team projects?
Teamwork is pivotal to what I do not just in my current position but in all the roles that I have held. Teamwork allows me to tap into the expertise of other subject matter experts, which helps me to save time and better strategize to solve problems. Teams are a repository of experiences and resources. The better the team and it's the members, the better the outcomes! I have been involved in team projects for my company that have allowed us to create a new cultural platform that was instrumental in helping us, a start-up company, to better communicate our vision and values and recognize our associates.

What words of wisdom do you have for future dietetics professionals?
Dare to be different! If you have an interest or a specific vision of where you see nutrition or dietetics going, be the pioneer. You will never know it all, so be open to learning from everyone in all disciplines and industries. Get involved and give back, whether to your community or as a mentor; it makes you not only a better person, but also a better professional!

Suggested Activities

1. Interview someone who is currently involved in a supervised practice experience or who has completed one recently. Ask the person about his or her experiences, including likes and dislikes about the supervised practice experience. Ask for his or her advice as you consider the application process.
2. Look at the list of core competencies for supervised practice for DTRs or RDNs on the Academy website. How do these competencies relate to the "Core Knowledge" acquired during the didactic process?
3. Study the verbs used in the core competency statements. What do these indicate about the job activities of entry-level dietetics professionals?
4. Talk to someone who has just finished the supervised practice experience. Ask the individual to describe one of the best learning experiences and explain why the experience was so meaningful. What was a difficult learning experience, and what did the person bring away from that experience?
5. Complete a self-assessment plan.
   a. Go to the Academy website or look at a copy of the *Applicant Guide to Supervised Practice Experiences*, and identify three supervised practice programs in which you might be interested.
   b. Find out as much as you can about the supervised practice program through its webpage, printed material, or by contacting the program director for more information. Complete a written summary of each of the supervised practice programs. Make sure to include the following information:
      i. Number of students/interns applying
      ii. Number of applicants accepted in the last 2 years

       iii. Minimum GPA required

       iv. Average GPA of current students

       v. Length of the supervised practice program

       vi. Full-time program or part-time options?

       vii. What rotations are included in the program, where are the training sites, and how long are the rotations?

       viii. What is the cost of attending the program?

       ix. GRE required for admission?

       x. Option to obtain an advanced degree along with the supervised practice experience?

       xi. Other requirements for program admission, such as work experience or volunteer experience?

       xii. Interview required? If so, is it an in-person interview or a phone interview?

c. Summarize what these programs are looking for and how applicants are evaluated. Identify at least three criteria that are considered.

d. On each of these criteria, assess your own readiness on a scale of 1 to 10, with 1 being "needs a lot of work" and 10 being "outstanding."

e. Describe your readiness for the supervised practice experience, and justify the scores you gave yourself on the different criteria.

f. Design a plan and describe, in detail, what you can do to increase or maintain your scores so you can maximize your chances of being accepted into a supervised practice program.

Selected Websites

- www.dnddigital.com—D&D Digital.
- www.eatrightacend.org/ACEND/content.aspx?id=6442485414—Academy of Nutrition and Dietetics list of all accredited supervised practice programs.
- www.eatrightacend.org/ACEND/content.aspx?id=6442485424—Academy of Nutrition and Dietetics lists the DIs that operate by distance education.
- www.eatrightpro.org/resources/membership/student-member-center—Academy of Nutrition and Dietetics Student Center.
- www.eatright.org/uploadedFiles/CADE/CADE-General-Content/3-08_RD-FKC_Only.pdf—Competency statements for RDN programs.
- http://www.ndepnet.org/—Nutrition and Dietetics Educators and Preceptors.

References

1. Academy of Nutrition and Dietetics. 2012 ACEND Standards for Dietitian Education Programs. Available at: http://www.eatrightacend.org/ACEND/. Accessed January 12, 2016.

2. Academy of Nutrition and Dietetics. ACEND 2012 Standards for Technician Education Programs. Available at: http://www.eatrightacend.org/ACEND/. Accessed January 12, 2012.

3. Academy of Nutrition and Dietetics. Accredited Dietetic Education Programs. Available at: http://www.eatrightacend.org/ACEND/content.aspx?id=6442485414. Accessed January 12, 2016.

4. Academy of Nutrition and Dietetics. Percent Change in Number of Openings, Applicants, and Applicants Matched to DI Programs Participating in Computer Matching Process (April/November). Available at: http://www.eatrightacend.org/ACEND/content.aspx?id=6442485435. Accessed January 12, 2016.

5. Applicant Guide to Supervised Practice. Available at: http://www.eatrightstore.org/product/08F23664-C029-4116-9E37-E27713FED0A5. Accessed January 12, 2016.

6. Academy of Nutrition and Dietetics. Suggestions to Improve Your Chances at Getting a Dietetic Internship Position: Student Guidance Document. Available at: http://www.eatrightacend.org/ACEND/content.aspx?id=6442485432. Accessed March 20, 2016.

7. Academy of Nutrition and Dietetics. Dietetic Internships: Programs Offering Distance Education. Available at: http://www.eatrightacend.org/ACEND/content.aspx?id=6442485424. Accessed January 12, 2016.

8. Academy of Nutrition and Dietetics. Individualized Supervised Practice Pathways (ISPPs). http://www.eatrightacend.org/ACEND/content.aspx?id=6442485529. Accessed January 12, 2016.

9. Academy of Nutrition and Dietetics. Accredited Dietetics Education Programs. Available at: http://www.eatrightacend.org/ACEND/content.aspx?id=6442485414. Accessed January 12, 2016.

10. Academy of Nutrition and Dietetics. Dietetic Internships. Available at: http://www.eatrightacend.org/ACEND/content.aspx?id=6442485424. Accessed January 12, 2016.

11. Dietetic Internship Centralized Application System. Available at: http://link.videoplatform.limelight.com/media/?mediaId=231cab9211b341828ba1ce8edfa36b0d&width=1000&height=721&playerForm=845f85be3ed44f30a5c2b290f7871a6f. Accessed January 11, 2016.

12. D&D Digital. Available at: https://www.dnddigital.com/. Accessed January 12, 2016.

13. U.S. Department of Education. Family Educational Rights and Privacy Act (FERPA). Available at: http://www2.ed.gov/policy/gen/guid/fpco/ferpa/index.html. Accessed January 12, 2016.

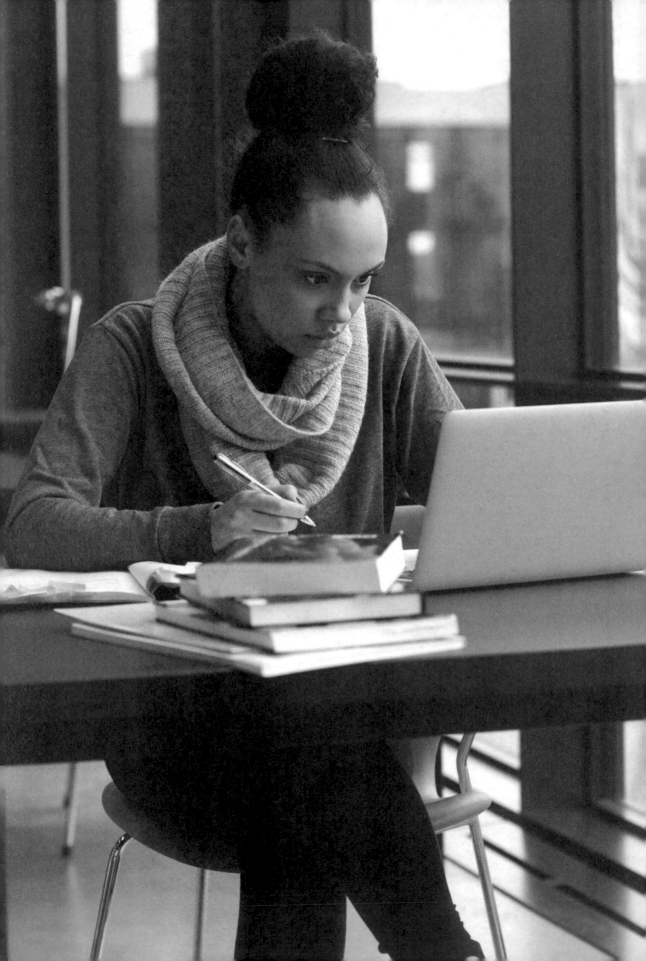

Credentialing

Protecting the Public

Defining the competence required of practitioners is an important quality assurance activity for any profession. According to *Webster's Dictionary*, the word *credential* means "a letter or certificate given to a person to show that he has a right to confidence or to the exercise of a certain position or authority; that which gives credit; that which entitles to credit, confidence, etc., establishing reliability."[1] This is an appropriate description of the work of the Commission on Dietetic Registration (CDR).

Commission on Dietetic Registration

The CDR, the credentialing arm of the Academy of Nutrition and Dietetics, was first called the Committee on Professional Registration. In 1969, it was charged with the implementation of national dietetic registration. In November 1975, the CDR was made an independent unit of the American Dietetic Association (ADA). The CDR is responsible for all aspects of the registration process: standard setting for registration eligibility, examination development and administration, credentialing, and recertification. The CDR grants recognition of entry-level competence to dietitians who meet its standards and qualifications. These dietitians may use the legally protected professional designation *Registered Dietitian* or *Registered Dietitian Nutritionist*, or the initials RD or RDN, respectively. Dietetic technicians who meet the standards and qualifications for technicians may use the legally protected professional designation *Dietetic Technician, Registered* or *Nutrition and Dietetics Technician, Registered*, or the initials DTR or NDTR, respectively.

The Commission consists of 11 members. Credentialed practitioners, RDNs and NDTRs, elect nine members. These include seven RDNs, one RDN specialist, and one NDTR. A newly credentialed practitioner is appointed by the Commission for a 1-year term. In addition, a public representative is appointed to the Commission and has full rights and privileges.[2]

Dietetic Registration

The purpose of registration is to protect the nutritional health, safety, and welfare of the public by encouraging high standards of performance of individuals practicing in the profession of dietetics.[3] Registration of dietitians began in 1969, providing a legally protected title for credentialed practitioners. At its inception, registration required membership in the ADA, completion of an examination, and a continuing education requirement. More than 19,000 members of the ADA were "grandfathered" and became registered during the initial enrollment period when the examination was waived.[3] As of June 14, 2016, there were 95,037 RDs/RDNs.[4] Dietetic technicians were first admitted to membership in the ADA in 1975. Certification for DTRs became a reality in 1983. The CDR currently recognizes 5,467 DTRs/NDTRs.[4] Membership in the Academy is not a requirement for RD/RDN or DTR/NDTR status.

The Registration Examination

The development of the examinations for RD/RDN and DTR/NDTR status is rigorous. **Figure 7–1** outlines the steps in the CDR's test development program.

The **dietetics practice audit** is the important first step in this process. A practice audit is an in-depth study of dietetics practice that describes the knowledge and skills needed to perform in a competent manner at a specified level of dietetics practice.

From the practice audit, a blueprint for building the examination must be developed. **Test specifications** include a description of the content to be tested, the proportion of the test to be devoted to various content areas, and the characteristics of acceptable test items. Because the test specifications come from the dietetics practice audit, the test is deemed to be valid and credible.

Test item development is an exciting but time-consuming experience. Individuals trained in the specifics of test construction develop test questions. Care is taken in choosing individuals who represent diverse practice areas and population subgroups. Four criteria are applied to each test question: (1) the question must be relevant and critical to entry-level practice; (2) the question must be accurate, current, and clear; (3) the question must not reflect regional or institutional differences; and (4) the question must conform to test specifications. Test items are reviewed by professional test editors to eliminate technical flaws, ambiguities, and potential bias. Questions that are considered to be editorially and technically sound are then pretested as unscored items on an actual exam. Such a "trial run" of the unscored items allows the test developers to see whether the test item truly discriminates between those who are entry-level competent and those who are not.

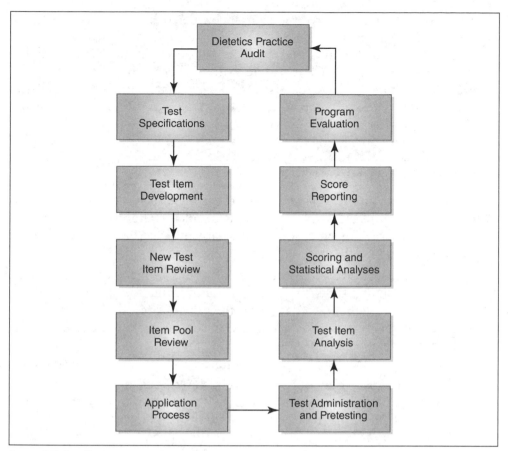

FIGURE 7–1 Certification testing program.
Courtesy of Commission on Dietetic Registration, Academy of Nutrition and Dietetics, Chicago, IL

During the **item pool review** process, experienced test reviewers appointed by the CDR review the items for content accuracy, currency, and relevance to entry-level practice. They must also be sure that each item has one best answer. Only when a test item has successfully passed the content, measurement, and editorial review will that item be included in the computer-based test item pool.

After each test item has been pretested as an unscored item, psychometricians perform **test item analysis**. Performance statistics are reviewed for each test question to identify problems. Experienced item writers review test items that appear to be problematic before those items are included in the scored item pool. This eliminates items with potential response problems or ambiguities. This review process is repeated on an ongoing basis as test items are administered.

The CDR periodically conducts a **passing-score determination study**, using experienced dietetics professionals from diverse practice areas and population subgroups. Content experts establish the minimum level of acceptable professional performance expected on a certification test. The CDR uses a criterion-referenced approach for determining the passing score. This criterion-referenced passing score becomes the basis for equating future exams, thus ensuring that all the versions of the examinations are of equal level of difficulty.

Score reporting announces the examinee's performance on the certification exam. The report gives a total scaled score as well as subscaled scores in the different test domains (nutrition and foodservice). Twice a year, in February and August, the CDR provides dietetic education programs with both a test summary of how the institution's graduates have performed and also individual scores by name when the examinee has authorized his or her scores to be released to the program.[5]

Computer-Adaptive Testing

Since July 1999 computers have administered registration examinations for both RDs/RDNs and DTRs/NDTRs. CDR decided to implement computerized testing because it recognized the many advantages this method offers to examinees. These include the following:

- Flexible test administration dates allow examinees to schedule the examination at a time convenient to them throughout the year.
- Retesting is available 45 days after the previous test date.
- A unique examination is generated based on each examinee's entry-level competence.
- Score reports are distributed to examinees as they leave the test site.

The registration examinations are administered at Pearson-VUE test centers nationwide. Eligible candidates must use the Pearson-VUE web portal to schedule their reservation to take the examination. The cost is $200 for the *Registration Examination for Dietitian Nutritionists* and $120 for the *Registration Examination for Nutrition and Dietetics Technicians*.

The examinations are variable in length. For the RDN examination, each test taker is given a *minimum* of 125 questions; 100 of these are scored questions and 25 are questions that are being pretested for use on subsequent examinations and are unscored. The *maximum* number of questions possible is 145; 120 are scored questions and 25 are unscored pretest questions.

For the NDTR examination, each examinee is given a *minimum* of 110 questions; 80 of these are scored questions and 30 are unscored pretest questions. The *maximum* number of questions is 130, with 100 scored items and 30 unscored pretest items. All questions for either the RDN or NDTR exam are in multiple-choice format.

For both examinations, test takers are given a total of 3 hours, which includes time for an introductory tutorial. The clock starts ticking with the administration of the first test question. From that point, the test taker has a maximum of 2.5 hours to finish the exam. The test taker has the option of having the "time remaining" show on the screen. If watching those numbers click down is a distraction, you can hide the clock!

If you've never taken a computer-based examination, you should practice taking such a test. Note that on the computerized examination once a question is presented you must answer that question. You cannot skip to the next question or go back and change an answer. You must answer each question as it comes and then move to the next one.

The CDR has prepared two study guides, one for the RD/RDN exam and one for the DTR/NDTR exam. Both guides provide a comprehensive study outline, references, and a practice examination. A practice exam is available in both the printed and online versions of the study guide. The practice examination in the online version simulates the actual computerized registration examination format. You may purchase the study guides from the Academy by calling 1-800-877-1600, ext. 5000. Alternatively, you may purchase the study guides by visiting the Academy's eatright.store online (see http://www .eatrightstore.org/). The cost of either study guide is $65.

Individuals who have completed both the academic preparation and the supervised practice requirements and have received signed Verification Statements for both of these experiences may sit for the national *Registration Examination for Dietitian Nutritionists* or the *Registration Examination for Nutrition and Dietetics Technicians*. A Verification Statement signed by the program director and a transcript documenting completion of the required courses must be submitted with the examination application. If a person is returning to college or university to complete a degree started at some earlier time, a dietetics program may require that person to update previous coursework before issuing a Verification Statement. You should check with the dietetics program director to find out about such program requirements. Once your eligibility to take the examination has been established, you will be sent a letter that authorizes you to schedule an examination time with Pearson-VUE. This authorization document expires 1 year after its issuance. If you don't successfully complete the RD/RDN or DTR/NDTR exam within 1 year, you must contact CDR to be reauthorized.[5]

Getting Ready for the Credentialing Examination

The credentialing exam is the culmination of all your years of hard work and study. Preparing to take the exam can be a stressful time, and the examination may come at a very busy time. Perhaps you've just graduated or finished your supervised practice experience. Perhaps you're starting a new job, or you've just moved or gotten married or any other of the many life-changing experiences that may be happening as you move into your career. Finding time to organize and review your material may be a challenge, but it is a critical activity! No one should ever walk into the credentialing examination without lots of study and preparation.

As mentioned in the previous section, the CDR produces study guides for both the RD/RDN and DTR/NDTR examinations, and these publications are an excellent place to start the review process. However, you may wish to pursue other study activities. Several entrepreneurs have established workshops that help individuals organize and review for the RDN exam. Some of these also have printed study materials that are included in the registration fee to attend the workshop. Some sell these materials separately for study on your own. These RD/RDN exam review sessions may last 2 to 3 days and are held in various parts of the country. Check with your program director or look in the *Journal of the Academy of Nutrition and Dietetics* for further information. Examples include the reviews by Breeding & Associates[6] or Inman

Seminars.[7] Program directors are often contacted about these review sessions and can share this information with you. Some dietetic education programs also provide review sessions for their own graduates, and your program director will let you know if this service is available.

Other entrepreneurs have developed other media to help examinees study for the credentialing exam. Two examples are "RD in a Flash" flash cards[8] and DietitianExam.com, an online study program.[9] Before you pay for any kind of review material or program, ask the following questions to help you make a more informed decision:

- How long have you been in business?
- How many people have used your service?
- What is the pass rate on the RD/RDN exam of those people who have used your service?
- Would you share with me some names and contact information of individuals who have used your service?
- When did you last update your review materials?
- Do you have simulated computer-based testing as part of your service?

Taking the credentialing examination is a stressful experience. Before the scheduled time for your examination, keep the following in mind:

- Get a good night's sleep the night before the exam.
- Confirm the time and location of the exam.
- Allow yourself plenty of time to get to the testing site. If you do not arrive on time, the test will have to be rescheduled.
- Make sure you arrive with a photo ID for identification purposes.
- A calculator will be provided for you at the test site. Don't try taking your own; you won't be allowed to use it.
- If you encounter a computer malfunction during the exam, you will be asked to wait 45 minutes while the problem is investigated. If it is not possible to resolve the problem in this time frame, you will be rescheduled to retest as soon as possible.
- Remember, if you don't pass the exam, it's not the end of the world! You may retake the exam as soon as 45 days later. Review your materials and try again.
- When you pass, celebrate by sharing the good news with your didactic program director and your supervised practice program director.

Maintaining Registered Status

Continuing education has always been an integral part of professional registration. As the profession of dietetics continues to change and expand into new areas of practice, it is vital that dietetics professionals be lifelong learners. As we move into new and uncharted waters, each of us must update and broaden our knowledge base for effective dietetics practice. CDR was one of the first health-related credentialing agencies to insist on continuing education. To maintain registered status, dietetics professionals must document their participation in professional development activities by creating a Professional Development Portfolio (PDP). During each 5-year reporting period, RDs/RDNs must achieve 75 continuing professional education units (CPEUs), and DTRs/NDTRs must achieve 50 CPEUs. The CPEUs must be based on each person's individual learning needs as identified in the professional development portfolio process.

Steps in Professional Portfolio Development

The steps in developing one's portfolio are as follows:

- Reflect on your professional practice to establish professional goals.
- Conduct a learning needs assessment to identify what you know now and what you need to learn to reach your goals.
- Develop a learning plan that shows how you will meet your goals.
- Implement your learning plan through continuing professional development activities.
- Evaluate your learning plan outcomes to assess how you have applied what you've learned and its impact on reaching your goals, refocusing those goals when necessary.

The CDR defines *continuing education* as education beyond that required for entry into the profession. Educational programs may apply directly to the field of nutrition and dietetics, or they may launch the learner into new areas such as computer technology, physical assessment, or marketing. Whatever the learning activity, it should update or enhance one's knowledge and skills for new applications in dietetics practice. Some examples of continuing education activities include:

- Lectures
- Workshops
- Journal clubs and study groups
- Seminars
- Case presentations
- Video, audio, and computer-based materials
- Self-study programs
- Culinary skills training
- Physical assessment training
- Multiskill training
- Computer technology training

Take a few minutes to watch the PDP Tutorial Presentation on the CDR website for more detailed information about the PDP process.[10]

Specialty Credentials

In 1993, the first specialty examinations were administered, enabling RDs who met the prescribed criteria to become board certified in specific specialty areas of dietetics practice. Currently, the CDR offers specialty credentials in five areas:

- Board Certified Specialist in Renal Nutrition (CSR)
- Board Certified Specialist in Pediatric Nutrition (CSP)
- Board Certified Specialist in Sports Dietetics (CSSD)

- Board Certified Specialist in Gerontological Nutrition (CSG)
- Board Certified Specialist in Oncology Nutrition (CSO)

These credentials typically require that the candidate has been an RD/RDN for at least 2 years and have from 1,500 to 2,000 hours of practice in the area of specialty. The schedules of when and where examinations will be administered are announced each year by CDR. Criteria for eligibility to sit for the examinations and other details about each credential may be found online at www.cdrnet.org/certifications.[11] As of June 14, 2015, there were 648 CSRs, 975 CSPs, 788 CSSDs, 606 CSGs, and 694 CSOs.[12]

Specialty credentials are also available from other professional organizations. Some of these certifications are listed in **Table 7–1**.

TABLE 7–1

Health- and Fitness-Related Credentials

Credential	Contact Information
ACE Certified Clinical Exercise Specialist	American Council on Exercise 4851 Paramount Drive, San Diego, CA 92123 Phone: 800-825-3636 Email: support@acefitness.org
ACE Certified Group Fitness Instructor	American Council on Exercise 4851 Paramount Drive, San Diego, CA 92123 Phone: 800-825-3636 Email: support@acefitness.org
ACE Certified Lifestyle & Weight Management Consultant	American Council on Exercise 4851 Paramount Drive, San Diego, CA 92123 Phone: 800-825-3636 Email: support@acefitness.org
ACE Certified Personal Trainer	American Council on Exercise 4851 Paramount Drive, San Diego, CA 92123 Phone: 800-825-3636 Email: support@acefitness.org
ACSM Certified Exercise Specialist Instructor	American College of Sports Medicine P.O. Box 1440 Indianapolis, IN 46206-1440 Phone: 317-637-9200 Email: certification@acsm.org
ACSM Certified Health/Fitness Instructor	American College of Sports Medicine P.O. Box 1440 Indianapolis, IN 46206-1440 Phone: 317-637-9200 Email: certification@acsm.org
ACSM Registered Clinical Exercise Physiologist	American College of Sports Medicine P.O. Box 1440 Indianapolis, IN 46206-1440 Phone: 317-637-9200 Email: certification@acsm.org
Board Certified in Advanced Diabetes Management	American Association of Diabetes Educators 200 W. Madison Street, Suite 800 Chicago, IL 60606 Phone: 800-338-3633

Certified Clinical Nutritionist (CCN)	International and American Associations of Clinical Nutritionists (IAACN) 15280 Addison Road, Suite 130 Addison, TX 75001 Phone: 972-407-9089
Certified Diabetes Educator (CDE)	National Certification Board for Diabetes Educators 330 E. Algonquin Road, Suite 4 Arlington Heights, IL 60005 Phone: 847-228-9795
Certified in Family and Consumer Sciences (CFCS)	American Association of Family and Consumer Sciences 400 N. Columbus Street, Suite 202 Alexandria, VA 22314 Phone: 703-706-4600
Certified Foodservice Professional (CFSP)	North American Association of Food Equipment Manufacturers 161 N. Clark Street, Suite 2020 Chicago, IL 60601 Phone: 312-821-0201
Certified Health Education Specialist (CHES)	National Commission for Health Education Credentialing, Inc. 1541 Alta Drive, Suite 303 Whitehall, PA 18052-5642 Phone: 800-813-0727
Certified Nutrition Specialist (CNS)	Certification Board of Nutrition Specialists of the American College of Nutrition 300 S. Duncan Avenue, Suite 225 Clearwater, FL 33755 Phone: 727-446-6086
Certified Nutrition Support Clinician (CNSC)	National Board of Nutrition Support Certification, Inc., of the American Society for Parenteral and Enteral Nutrition 8630 Fenton Street, Suite 412 Silver Spring, MD 20910 Phone: 301-587-6315 or 800-727-4567
Certified Professional in Healthcare Quality	Healthcare Quality Certification Board of the National Association for Healthcare Quality 18000 W. 105th Street Olathe, KS 66061-7543 Phone: 913-895-4609
International Board Certified Lactation Consultant, Registered Lactation Consultant (IBCLC, RLC)	International Board of Lactation Consultant Examiners 6402 Arlington Boulevard, Suite 350 Falls Church, VA 22042 Phone: 703-560-7330
National Certified Counselor	National Board for Certified Counselors 3 Terrace Way, Suite D Greensboro, NC 27403-3660 Phone: 336-547-0607
School Foodservice and Nutrition Specialist (SFNS)	School Nutrition Association 700 S. Washington Street, Suite 300 Alexandria, VA 22314 Phone: 703-739-3900

Specialty credentials can be a valuable asset to the dietitian who holds them. Career advancement may be enhanced, salary levels may increase, and recognition of heightened expertise by other members of the healthcare team may be realized.

Fellow of the American Dietetic Association/Fellow of the Academy of Nutrition and Dietetics

The ADA established the credential *Fellow* to certify those registered dietitians who demonstrated empirically defined characteristics of achievement and leadership (abbreviated FADA, for Fellow of the ADA). To become a FADA, candidates had to meet the following requirements:

- Be an RD.
- Submit documentation of a minimum of a master's degree, earned and granted by a regionally accredited U.S. college or university or foreign equivalent.
- Submit documentation of a minimum of 8 years of work experience as an RD.
- Submit documentation of at least one professional achievement.
- Submit documentation of professional positions.
- Submit documentation of professional contacts.
- Submit a written response to an approach-to-practice scenario.

A portfolio submitted by the candidate was judged through peer review. Certification as a FADA was granted for a 10-year period. During that period, fellows were required to maintain RD status and submit an annual maintenance fee. At this time, CDR is not accepting new applications for the FADA credential. However, you may meet RDs who have earned the FADA designation and continue to use this credential after their name.[13] Recommendation 8 in the "Final Report of the Phase 2 Future Practice and Education Task Force" has recommended the reinstitution of an advanced-level practice credential in the future.[14]

The Academy has now established a Fellow of the Academy of Nutrition and Dietetics, or FAND, program to "recognize Academy members who have distinguished themselves among their colleagues, as well as in their communities, by their service to the dietetics profession and by optimizing the nation's health through food and nutrition."[15] A Fellow is expected to embody the Academy's values of customer focus, integrity, innovation, and social responsibility. Further information about the FAND designation may be found on the Academy website.[15]

Licensure

Licensure is "a state policy that provides consumers an assurance that a professional is competent to provide certain services and is used by professionals to exclude the non-licensed from providing those services for a fee. It is a tool for creating and maintaining a verifiable minimum level of skill and competence."[16]

Licensure differs from registration in several ways. Although registration is recognized nationally, licensure is recognition by an individual state. Both credentialing systems afford some legal protection to the title of the practitioner, but licensure may also protect the right of an individual to practice in a state. Registration is voluntary, established and maintained in the private sector. Licensure may be either voluntary or mandatory, but it has formal legal status in the public sector.

At present, 45 states, the District of Columbia, and Puerto Rico have enacted some form of regulation. **Licensing statutes** include an explicitly defined scope of practice and make it illegal to practice dietetics without first obtaining a license from the state. **Statutory certification** limits the use of particular titles to persons meeting predetermined requirements, but persons not certified can still practice dietetics with a different title. **Registration** is the least restrictive form of state regulation. It prohibits use of the title *dietitian* by those not meeting state-mandated qualifications. However, unregistered persons may practice the profession.

Each state has a licensure contact person who can provide updates on professional regulation in that state. The name and telephone number of any state's licensure contact can be found on the CDR website (www.cdrnet.org).[17]

As you ready to enter dietetics practice, be sure to check the CDR list to find out about the status of licensure in the state where you plan on living and starting your career. Call the contact person listed and ask any questions you might have.

It is possible that you may be hired on a probationary basis as an entry-level dietitian before you have taken and passed the RD/RDN examination. In states that have licensure, the RD/RDN exam is considered "the licensure exam" and proof of readiness for practice If you have not yet taken the RD/RDN examination by the time you start your first job, you may be granted a temporary license to practice in the state for a limited time until you pass the exam. Be sure to discuss all of these issues with both prospective employers and the licensing board in your proposed state of residence.

Other Tools Supporting Professional Competence

Evidence-Based Practice

According to the Academy, *evidence-based practice* is "the use of systematically reviewed scientific evidence in making food and nutrition practice decisions by integrating best available evidence with professional expertise and client values to improve outcomes."[18] The Academy has developed a plethora of resources to help dietetics professionals make practice decisions based on the best available scientific evidence. This evidence researches findings as well as national guidelines, policies, consensus statements, expert opinions, and quality improvement data.[18]

One of the most outstanding resources is the Academy's Evidence Analysis Library®. This resource, which is available free to Academy members, is a synthesis of the best, most relevant nutritional research on important dietetic practice questions in an accessible, online, user-friendly library.[19] The library covers a wide variety of topics including childhood overweight and obesity, nutritional counseling, critical illness, and so on. The database is consistently being updated and is available to members at any time.

Integrating research into daily dietetics practice is another important aspect of evidence-based practice. Dietetics professionals not only need to be informed of research going on in medical centers, universities, and so on, but also recognize that they can participate in research as part of their own dietetics practice. The Dietetics Practice-Based Research Network (DPBRN) brings together dietetics practitioners and researchers to identify and design research that can be carried out on the job.[20] Dietitians can propose ideas for research projects, serve on the advisory board that selects research projects to be pursued, help collect data on the job, and be a part of disseminating the research findings. You can find out more about the DPBRN on the Academy's website (www.eatright.org).

Standards of Practice and Standards of Professional Performance

The Standards of Practice (SOPs) and Standards of Professional Performance (SOPPs) are tools for credentialed dietetics practitioners to use in professional development. They serve as guides for self-evaluation and to determine the education and skills needed to advance an individual's level of practice. Although not regulations, the standards may be used by regulatory agencies to determine competency for credentialed dietetics practitioners.[21] The "American Dietetic Association Revised 2008 Standards of Practice in Nutrition Care and Standards of Professional Performance for Registered Dietitians and Dietetic Technicians, Registered" was published in the September 2008 issue of the *Journal of the American Dietetic Association*. These standards outline the minimum competent levels of practice for RDs/RDNs and DTRs/NDTRs and serve as the core statements of professional competency. From this core, practice-specific SOPs and SOPPs have been developed. These practice-specific standards may be viewed on the Academy website (www.eatright.org).

The SOPs relate directly to patient care and are based on the four steps of the Nutrition Care Process (NCP):

- Nutrition Assessment
- Nutrition Diagnosis
- Nutrition Intervention
- Nutrition Monitoring and Evaluation

The SOPPs represent six domains of professionalism:

- Provision of Services
- Application of Research
- Communication and Application of Knowledge
- Utilization and Management of Resources
- Quality in Practice
- Competency and Accountability[22]

The SOPs and SOPPs are designed to be used for self-evaluation and can be used as part of the Professional Development Portfolio as each dietetic practitioner strives for ever-increasing levels of competence in his or her practice.

The Code of Ethics for the Profession of Dietetics

This enforceable code provides for public accountability by monitoring appropriate ethical performance by a dietetics practitioner and reflects the individual's responsibility for competence in practice. The ADA Code of Ethics Task Force reviewed and revised the 1999 Code of Ethics in March 2009, and the ADA Board of Directors, the CDR, and the House of Delegates approved it in May 2009. The 2009 Code of Ethics was published in August 2009 in the *Journal of the American Dietetic Association* (pp. 1461–1467). The 2009 Code has been in effect as of January 1, 2010, and the 1999 version of the code is no longer valid.[23]

The current code of ethics (see **Figure 7–2**) outlines ethics considerations in four areas: (1) responsibilities to the public, (2) responsibilities to clients, (3) responsibilities to the profession, and (4) responsibilities to colleagues and other professionals. Although the Code applies to all RDs/RDNs and DTRs/NDTRs, discussing ethics in different practice settings helps dietetics practitioners to conceptualize ethical dilemmas they may face in their own practice.

PREAMBLE

The Academy of Nutrition and Dietetics and its credentialing agency, the Commission on Dietetic Registration (CDR), believe it is in the best interest of the profession and the public it serves to have a Code of Ethics in place that provides guidance to dietetics practitioners in their professional practice and conduct. Dietetics practitioners have voluntarily adopted this Code of Ethics to reflect the values and ethical principles guiding the dietetics profession and to set forth commitments and obligations of the dietetics practitioner to the public, clients, the profession, colleagues, and other professionals. The current Code of Ethics was approved on June 2, 2009, by the ADA Board of Directors, House of Delegates, and the Commission on Dietetic Registration.

APPLICATION

The Code of Ethics applies to the following practitioners: (a) In its entirety to members of the Academy who are Registered Dietitians (RDs) or Dietetic Technicians, Registered (DTRs); (b) Except for sections dealing solely with the credential, to all members of the Academy who are not RDs or DTRs; and (c) Except for aspects dealing solely with membership, to all RDs and DTRs who are not members of the Academy.

All individuals to whom the Code applies are referred to as "dietetics practitioners," and all such individuals who are RDs and DTRs shall be known as "credentialed practitioners." By accepting membership in to the Academy and/or accepting and maintaining CDR credentials, all members of the Academy and credentialed dietetics practitioners agree to abide by the Code.

PRINCIPLES

Fundamental Principles

1. The dietetics practitioner conducts himself/herself with honesty, integrity, and fairness.

FIGURE 7–2 Academy of Nutrition and Dietetics Code of Ethics. *(continues)*

2. The dietetics practitioner supports and promotes high standards of professional practice. The dietetics practitioner accepts the obligation to protect clients, the public, and the profession by upholding the Code of Ethics for the Profession of Dietetics and by reporting perceived violations of the Code through the processes established by the Academy and its credentialing agency, CDR.

Responsibilities to the Public

3. The dietetics practitioner considers the health, safety, and welfare of the public at all times. The dietetics practitioner will report inappropriate behavior or treatment of a client by another dietetics practitioner or other professionals.
4. The dietetics practitioner complies with all laws and regulations applicable or related to the profession or to the practitioner's ethical obligations as described in this Code.
   a. The dietetics practitioner must not be convicted of a crime under the laws of the United States, whether a felony or a misdemeanor, an essential element of which is dishonesty.
   b. The dietetics practitioner must not be disciplined by a state for conduct that would violate one or more of these principles.
   c. The dietetics practitioner must not commit an act of misfeasance or malfeasance that is directly related to the practice of the profession as determined by a court of competent jurisdiction, a licensing board, or an agency of a governmental body.
5. The dietetics practitioner provides professional services with objectivity and with respect for the unique needs and values of individuals.
   a. The dietetics practitioner does not, in professional practice, discriminate against others on the basis of race, ethnicity, creed, religion, disability, gender, age, gender identity, sexual orientation, national origin, economic status, or any other legally protected category.
   b. The dietetics practitioner provides services in a manner that is sensitive to cultural differences.
   c. The dietetics practitioner does not engage in sexual harassment in connection with professional practice.
6. The dietetics practitioner does not engage in false or misleading practices or communications.
   a. The dietetics practitioner does not engage in false or deceptive advertising of his or her services.
   b. The dietetics practitioner promotes or endorses specific goods or products only in a manner that is not false and misleading.
   c. The dietetics practitioner provides accurate and truthful information in communicating with the public.
7. The dietetics practitioner withdraws from professional practice when unable to fulfill his or her professional duties and responsibilities to clients and others.
   a. The dietetics practitioner withdraws from practice when he/she has engaged in abuse of a substance such that it could affect his or her practice.
   b. The dietetics practitioner ceases practice when he or she has been adjudged by a court to be mentally incompetent.
   c. The dietetics practitioner will not engage in practice when he or she has a condition that substantially impairs his or her ability to provide effective service to others.

FIGURE 7–2 Academy of Nutrition and Dietetics Code of Ethics. *(continued)*
Courtesy of Commission on Dietetic Registration, Academy of Nutrition and Dietetics, Chicago, IL

Responsibilities to Clients

8. The dietetics practitioner recognizes and exercises professional judgment within the limits of his or her qualifications and collaborates with others, seeks counsel, or makes referrals as appropriate.
9. The dietetics practitioner treats clients and patients with respect and consideration.
    a. The dietetics practitioner provides sufficient information to enable clients and others to make their own informed decisions.
    b. The dietetics practitioner respects the client's right to make decisions regarding the recommended plan of care, including consent, modification, or refusal.
10. The dietetics practitioner protects confidential information and makes full disclosure about any limitations on his or her ability to guarantee full confidentiality.
11. The dietetics practitioner, in dealing with and providing services to clients and others, complies with the same principles set forth above in "Responsibilities to the Public" (Principles #3–7).

Responsibilities to the Profession

12. The dietetics practitioner practices dietetics based on evidence-based principles and current information.
13. The dietetics practitioner presents reliable and substantiated information and interprets controversial information without personal bias, recognizing that legitimate differences of opinion exist.
14. The dietetics practitioner assumes a life-long responsibility and accountability for personal competence in practice, consistent with accepted professional standards, continually striving to increase professional knowledge and skills and to apply them in practice.
15. The dietetics practitioner is alert to the occurrence of a real or potential conflict of interest and takes appropriate action whenever a conflict arises.
    a. The dietetics practitioner makes full disclosure of any real or perceived conflict of interest.
    b. When a conflict of interest cannot be resolved by disclosure, the dietetics practitioner takes such other action as may be necessary to eliminate the conflict, including recusal from an office, position, or practice situation.
16. The dietetics practitioner permits the use of his or her name for the purpose of certifying that dietetics services have been rendered only if he or she has provided or supervised the provision of those services.
17. The dietetics practitioner accurately presents professional qualifications and credentials.
    a. The dietetics practitioner, in seeking, maintaining, and using credentials provided by CDR, provides accurate information and complies with all requirements imposed by CDR. The dietetics practitioner uses CDR-awarded credentials ("RD" or "Registered Dietitian"; "DTR" or "Dietetic Technician, Registered"; "CS" or "Certified Specialist"; and "FADA" or "Fellow of the American Dietetic Association") only when the credential is current and authorized by CDR.
    b. The dietetics practitioner does not aid any other person in violating any CDR requirements, or in representing him or herself as CDR-credentialed when he or she is not.
18. The dietetics practitioner does not invite, accept, or offer gifts, monetary incentives, or other considerations that affect or reasonably give an appearance of affecting his/her professional judgment.

FIGURE 7–2 Academy of Nutrition and Dietetics Code of Ethics. *(continued)*
Courtesy of Commission on Dietetic Registration, Academy of Nutrition and Dietetics, Chicago, IL

Clarification of Principle:

a. Whether a gift, incentive, or other item of consideration shall be viewed to affect, or give the appearance of affecting, a dietetics practitioner's professional judgment is dependent on all factors relating to the transaction, including the amount or value of the consideration, the likelihood that the practitioner's judgment will or is intended to be affected, the position held by the practitioner, and whether the consideration is offered or generally available to persons other than the practitioner.

b. It shall not be a violation of this principle for a dietetic compensation as a consultant or employee or as part of a research grant or corporate sponsorship program, provided the relationship is openly disclosed and the practitioner acts with integrity in performing the services or responsibilities.

c. This principle shall not preclude a dietetics practitioner from accepting gifts of nominal value, attendance at educational programs, meals in connection with educational exchanges of information, free samples of products, or similar items, as long as such items are not offered in exchange for or with the expectation of, and do not result in, conduct or services that are contrary to the practitioner's professional judgment.

d. The test for appearance of impropriety is whether the conduct would create in reasonable minds a perception that the dietetics practitioner's ability to carry out professional responsibilities with integrity, impartiality, and competence is impaired.

Responsibilities to Colleagues and Other Professionals

19. The dietetics practitioner demonstrates respect for the values, rights, knowledge, and skills of colleagues and other professionals.

a. The dietetics practitioner does not engage in dishonest, misleading, or inappropriate business practices that demonstrate a disregard for the rights or interests of others.

b. The dietetics practitioner provides objective evaluations of performance for employees and coworkers, candidates for employment, students, professional association memberships, awards, or scholarships, making all reasonable efforts to avoid bias in the professional evaluation of others.

Figure 7–2 Academy of Nutrition and Dietetics Code of Ethics.
Courtesy of Commission on Dietetic Registration, Academy of Nutrition and Dietetics, Chicago, IL

The Code of Ethics also outlines the process for consideration of ethics issues and how ethics cases are handled. Disciplinary actions may be taken against a dietetics practitioner who is found to be in violation of the Code of Ethics. Disciplinary actions may include censure, probation, suspension of Academy membership, suspension of registration, expulsion from membership, or revocation of registration status.[23]

The Code of Ethics section of the Academy website (www.eatright.org) offers a wealth of information about the Code and its applications. The site includes numerous educational resource links as well as a "Watch and Learn" video presentation about the Code and why it is important to dietetics professionals and the profession of dietetics.[23,24]

Summary

Each dietetic student should have the goal of becoming a credentialed dietetics practitioner. Although completion of an associate or baccalaureate degree in dietetics is a worthy achievement, earning the professional credential of DTR/NDTR or RD/RDN opens the doors for successful professional practice. This credential is your clients' assurance of your qualifications to practice, and it indicates that you actively work to update yourself on the latest information about food and nutrition issues. Licensure indicates that the state in which you practice recognizes your professional competence and expertise.

Specialty certification will become more common in the years ahead, as dietetics practice becomes increasingly complex and diverse. Professional credentialing is the mark of quality practice; it assures the public that the dietetic technician or registered dietitian is providing the highest quality in dietetics services.

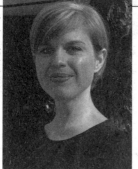

Courtesy of Petra Colindres

Profile of a Professional

Petra Colindres, MA, RDN/LD, IBCLC, CPT

Wellbeing Program Coordinator
State of Oklahoma, Oklahoma City, Oklahoma

Education:
BS in Advertising and Graphic Design, University of Central Oklahoma, Edmond, Oklahoma
MA in Nutritional Sciences, University of Oklahoma, Norman, Oklahoma

How did you first hear about dietetics and decide to become a Registered Dietitian?
I first heard about dietetics from my roommate. She was studying nutrition and considering going into the field. I was drawn to the profession immediately due to my interest in food, movement, and healthy family units.

What was your route to registration?
I graduated with honors from the University of Oklahoma Nutritional Sciences program. I was then accepted into their internship program and did 8 months of rotations through the University of Oklahoma Medical Center.

Where did you complete your supervised practice experience (if applicable)?
I completed a Dietetic Internship at University of Oklahoma Medical Center, Oklahoma City, Oklahoma.

Do you have an advanced degree(s)? If so, in what and from where?
I have my Master of Arts in Nutritional Sciences from University of Oklahoma. I also have a specialized board certification in lactation (International Board Certified Lactation Consultant), and I am a certified personal trainer through National Academy of Sports Medicine (NASM).

How have you been involved professionally?
I have been a member of the Academy for a number of years and am currently the president-elect for Oklahoma's local chapter. In addition to my involvement with nutrition organizations, I also currently serve as the vice president for the Oklahoma Lactation Consultant Association and as the communications co-chair for the Oklahoma Turning Point Council, a group created to transform public health in Oklahoma by working directly with community partnerships to improve health initiatives. I also

am a spokesperson for the American Heart Association, helping them identify food deserts in the state of Oklahoma and creating awareness to create healthy food choices for those affected. In the past, I have served as a board chair member for Infant Crisis Center, a nonprofit that serves to help infants at risk.

What honors or awards have you received?
I graduated with honors from my university and also received the Outstanding Didactic Program in Dietetics (DPD) Student Award from my university.

Briefly describe your career path in dietetics. What are you doing now?
My career first began in advertising and graphic design, where I spent approximately 2 years in the field. However, I quickly became fascinated with nutrition and realized that helping people create a healthier and happier life was my passion. This led me to changing my career and pursuing my graduate degree in Nutritional Sciences from the University of Oklahoma. Also, I decided to advance my degree by getting board certified in lactation. I seized the opportunity to focus my career on the family unit to instill positive lifestyle habits.

Today, I work with the State of Oklahoma as the State Well-Being Program Coordinator. The state is currently creating a more holistic approach to well-being that encompasses the entire person and includes the family as an approach to ensure healthy lifestyle habits. In my current position, I focus my efforts on creating change that helps mothers and families prepare for healthy futures in the workplace. This includes my work on issues from lactation support programs, nutrition recommendations and policies, training and development classes, and traditional programing. At the heart of what we do, our goal is to create an open culture in the workplace that allows well-being and health initiatives to thrive. My profession is great in that there's a lot of room to grow and no 2 days are ever the same. In addition, I have my own consulting practice that focuses on early childhood nutrition. Within my practice, I do pediatric counseling, lactation support, children's cooking classes, and local seminars around the state.

What excites you about dietetics and the future of our profession?
What excites me is the variety of jobs within our field. I use to believe that to be a "real" dietitian, you had to work either in a hospital or an outpatient setting. However, this is far from the truth! Growth within our field and the need in our country have created many jobs where a nutrition expert is of high importance.

How is teamwork important to you in your position? How have you been involved in team projects?
Teamwork and relationship building are integral parts of the job description. My job depends on resources and knowledge that I cannot accomplish by myself. To elaborate, our programming focuses on six areas of well-being (e.g., physical, financial, and emotional). Our team is a pod of four professionals with expertise in varying areas. I lean on my coworkers a lot for an integrated approach to our projects; I often joke that you would not want me to give anyone financial advice! Beyond that, as a state department, we work within our agencies to utilize resources. We see our employees as our best support for our programming, so we look to them for needs, interests, and collaboration. Part of our job is to break down the silos within the workplace and help create open communication between the agencies to increase engagement within the state. You cannot do that alone! Luckily, there's a lot of interest within agencies to partner to help create our overreaching goals.

What words of wisdom do you have for future dietetics professionals?
My words of wisdom would be to get involved in everything that interests you as a nutrition student. You never know where those connections will lead. My volunteering and blogging as a student led me to job opportunities that would have otherwise been closed off to me. Also, make a presence for yourself. Whether you blog, teach, or cook, become the local "it" person in your area for your specialty.

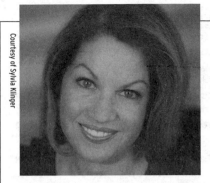

Courtesy of Sylvia Klinger

Profile of a Professional

Sylvia Klinger, DBA, RD

Nutrition and Culinary Consultant
Hispanic Food Communications, Washington, DC

Education:
BS in Nutrition and Dietetics with a major in
Administrative Dietetics, Loma Linda University,
Loma Linda, California
MS in Public Service Administration, DePaul
University, Chicago, Illinois

How did you first hear about dietetics and decide to become a Registered Dietitian?
My mom, who is an RD, played a significant role in my decision to become a dietitian.
But also some of my best friends lighted the passion for dietetics that was seeded by
my mom. While in high school, my best friends joined a new nutrition elective program offered at our high school. One afternoon as they were showing me their newly
created recipes and menus, I decided that this program was my cup of tea. I immediately joined the class, loved every minute, and have never looked back.

What was your route to registration?
I went to a coordinated program, which makes students eligible to take the RD exam
right after graduation. I loved my dietetics program, which prepared me to be the
best possible RD.

Where did you complete your supervised practice experience?
I graduated from a coordinated undergraduate program; therefore, my practicum
was completed at various facilities such as Loma Linda University Medical Center,
Loma Linda Veterans hospital, and a diabetic camp.

How have you been involved professionally?
I love my profession and was involved with the Academy of Nutrition and Dietetics
even before I graduated, so I have been involved with the Academy for more than
30 years! Here are some of my proud moments with the Academy:

- Currently Past Chair of Latinos and Hispanics in Dietetics and Nutrition Member
  Interest Group. Other positions held: Chair-Elect, Chair, Nominating Chair.
- Regional Coordinator for Dietitians in Business and Communications dietetics
  practice group.
- Most recently (12/30/2016), I authored a counseling kit with the Academy of Nutri-
  tion and Dietetics.

What honors or awards have you received?
In 1994, the Chicago Dietetic Association presented me with the Recognized Young
Dietitian of the Year award, and in 2009, I was awarded Outstanding Dietitian of the
Year. In 2012, I was honored to be awarded the Loma Linda University Distinguished
Alumna of the Year and the Rincon service award. Most recently, I received the 2013
Mujeres Destacadas Award by La Raza Newspaper.

Briefly describe your career path in dietetics. What are you doing now?
My career path started in management as that was my major while pursuing my
undergraduate degree in dietetics, but I quickly learned that in order to become more
marketable, you need a wide range of experiences. I started as a foodservice dietitian
at small hospital in New England (Massachusetts) followed by a few years working
for the Women, Infants, and Children (WIC) program, which became my springboard
to becoming an outpatient dietitian at the University of California Irvine Medical
Center. There I not only provided all of the counseling for most outpatient programs,
but also provided dietary counseling and research data collection for longitudinal

cardiovascular research. After a few years in the clinical setting, I moved to Chicago to pursue my graduate studies, but I was able to continue working with the same cardiovascular research at Northwestern Hospital preventive medicine research. After graduating with my master's degree, I landed an exciting corporate job with the Quaker Oats Company in Chicago, which lasted almost 10 years.

All of those amazing experiences gave me the courage and knowledge to launch my own consulting business, Hispanic Food Communications, through which I am very proud to advise companies and the public with science-based nutrition messages.

What excites you about dietetics and the future of our profession?
There is so much to be excited about in our profession as this is our moment to shine! With the current state of our population's health, I believe it is our responsibility to educate and motivate our people to start practicing simple healthy habits one step at a time. This huge responsibility motivates me every day to proudly continue my role in world of nutrition.

How is teamwork important to you in your position? How have you been involved in team projects?
Teamwork is everything to me. I can't do it alone; therefore, I value teamwork. I get excited when we are brainstorming ideas or working on projects together. The energy generated is contagious, and it helps us to keep the momentum going when it gets tough.

What words of wisdom do you have for future dietetics professionals?
I have learned a few things while going down my path: Attitude is everything, so keep it positive. Communicate well (which means communicate constantly) with your peers and managers, deliver more than you are required, and do it for the love of the game (your career)! I love nutrition! I love my career path! It's been a wonderful ride, and I owe everything to my family and friends who have supported me for the last few decades.

Suggested Activities

1. Talk to someone who has recently taken the registration examination for RDs/RDNs or DTRs/NDTRs. What was his or her reaction to the experience? What suggestions does he or she have for preparing for the exam?

2. Look in the back of the *Journal of the Academy of Nutrition and Dietetics* or go online and look at the RD/RDN exam review ads. What kinds of tools are available to help you prepare for the test? How much do they cost? What are some less expensive ways you could prepare for the credentialing exam?

3. Who is your state continuing education coordinator? If possible, talk to this person and find out what kinds of continuing education events he or she approves. What process must be followed to get an event approved for continuing education credit?

4. Attend a continuing education event with a dietetics professional, faculty member, or another student. What kind of documentation must be provided for an attendee to receive continuing education credits?

5. Find out if your state has licensure for dietitians. If so, work with your teacher to invite someone to your class to talk about licensure, what it means in your state, and how it was obtained in the legislature. What is the process for becoming licensed in your state?

6. Pick another professional credential besides the DTR/NDTR or RD/RDN that you might be interested in pursuing. Visit the website of the certifying agency and find out exactly what you would need to do to earn that credential or certification.
7. Talk with a dietetics professional about his or her career portfolio. Ask the professional to share with you what it was like to do self-assessment to determine continuing education goals. What kinds of continuing education opportunities has this person pursued to meet professional development goals?
8. What kind of continuing education requirements are there for other professional credentials? How do these requirements compare with dietetics requirements?

Selected Websites

- www.diabeteseducator.org—American Association of Diabetes Educators; offers information on the Board Certified in Advanced Diabetes Management (BC-ADM) credential.
- www.acsm.org—American College of Sports Medicine (ACSM); offers information on the various ACSM credentials.
- www.acefitness.org—American Council on Exercise (ACE); provides information on the various ACE credentials.
- www.eatright.org—Academy of Nutrition and Dietetics site offers purchase information for the *CDR RD Exam Study Guide* and the *CDR DTR Exam Study Guide*.
- www.cdrnet.org—CDR site offers information about CDR specialty credentials.
- www.dietitianexam.com—DietitianExam.com review program.
- www.iaacn.org—International and American Associations of Clinical Nutritionists; offers information on the Certified Clinical Nutritionist (CCN) credential.
- www.nafem.org—North American Association of Food Equipment Manufacturers; offers information on the Certified Foodservice Professional (CFSP) credential.
- www.ncbde.org—National Certification Board for Diabetes Educators; offers information on the Certified Diabetes Educator (CDE) credential.
- www.rdinaflash.com—"RD in a Flash" flash cards for RD exam review

References

1. *Webster's New Universal Unabridged Dictionary*, 2nd ed. New York: Simon & Schuster; 1983.
2. Commission on Dietetic Registration. Available at: https://www.cdrnet.org/about. Accessed January 14, 2016.
3. Woodward NM. The past, present, and future of dietetics credentialing. Future Search Conference: Challenging the Future of Dietetic Education and Credentialing. Background

Papers. Chicago: The American Dietetic Association and the Commission on Dietetic Registration, June 12–14, 1994.

4. Commission on Dietetic Registration. Registry Statistics. Available at: https://www.cdrnet.org/registry-statistics. Accessed April 25, 2016.

5. Commission on Dietetic Registration. Certification Testing Program. Available at: https://www.cdrnet.org/vault/2459/web/files/Excomponents.pdf. Accessed January 13, 2016.

6. Breeding & Associates Educational Resource Center. Available at: http://www.dietitianworkshops.com/. Accessed January 14, 2016.

7. Inman Seminars. Available at: http://www.inmanassoc.com. Accessed January 14, 2016.

8. RD in a Flash. Available at: http://www.rdinaflash.com. Accessed January 14, 2016.

9. DietitianExam.com. Available at: http://www.dietitianexam.com. Accessed January 14, 2016.

10. Commission on Dietetic Registration. Professional Development Portfolio Tutorial Presentation. Available at: https://www.cdrnet.org/pdp/commission-on-dietetic-registration-pdp-guide-tutorial-presentations. Accessed January 14, 2016.

11. Commission on Dietetic Registration. About CDR: Specialist Certification. Available at: https://www.cdrnet.org/about. Accessed January 14, 2016.

12. Commission on Dietetic Registration. Registry Statistics. Available at: https://www.cdrnet.org/registry-statistics. Accessed April 25, 2016.

13. Commission on Dietetic Registration. Fellow of the Academy of Nutrition and Dietetics. Available at: https://www.cdrnet.org/certifications/fellows-of-the-american-dietetic-association. Accessed March 22, 2016.

14. American Dietetic Association. Final Report of the Phase 2 Future Practice & Education Task Force. Available at: http://www.eatrightpro.org/~/media/eatrightpro%20files/practice/future%20practice/phase_2_future_practice_education_task_force_final_report.ashx. Accessed March 22, 2016.

15. Fellow of the Academy of Nutrition and Dietetics. Available at: http://www.eatrightpro.org/resource/membership/member-benefits/fellow-of-the-academy-of-nutrition-and-dietetics/fellow-of-the-academy-of-nutrition-and-dietetics. Accessed January 14, 2016.

16. Commission on Dietetic Registration. State Licensure. Available at: https://www.cdrnet.org/state-licensure. Accessed January 14, 2016.

17. Commission on Dietetic Registration. State Licensure Agency List. Available at: https://www.cdrnet.org/state-licensure-agency-list. Accessed January 14, 2016.

18. Academy of Nutrition and Dietetics. Evidence-Based Resources: Philosophy and Framework. Available at: http://www.eatrightpro.org/resources/research/evidence-based-resources/philosophy-and-framework. Accessed January 14, 2016.

19. Evidence Analysis Library. Available at: http://www.eatrightpro.org/resources/research/evidence-based-resources/evidence-analysis-library. Accessed January 14, 2016.

20. Academy of Nutrition and Dietetics. Dietetics Practice-Based Research Network. Available at: http://www.eatrightpro.org/resources/research/evidence-based-resources/dpbrn. Accessed January 14, 2016.

21. Academy of Nutrition and Dietetics. Practice Tips. Standards of Practice and Professional Performance. Available at: http://www.eatrightpro.org/resources/practice/quality-management/standards-of-practice. Accessed January 15, 2016.

22. Academy of Nutrition and Dietetics. Nutrition Care Process. Available at: http://www.eatrightpro.org/resources/practice/nutrition-care-process. Accessed January 15, 2016.

23. Academy of Nutrition and Dietetics. Ethics Education Resources. Available at: http://www.eatrightpro.org/resources/career/code-of-ethics/ethics-education-resources. Accessed January 15, 2016.

24. American Dietetic Association/Commission on Dietetic Registration. Code of ethics for the profession of dietetics and process for consideration of ethics issues. *J Am Diet Assoc.* 2009;109:1461–1467.

Professional Organizations

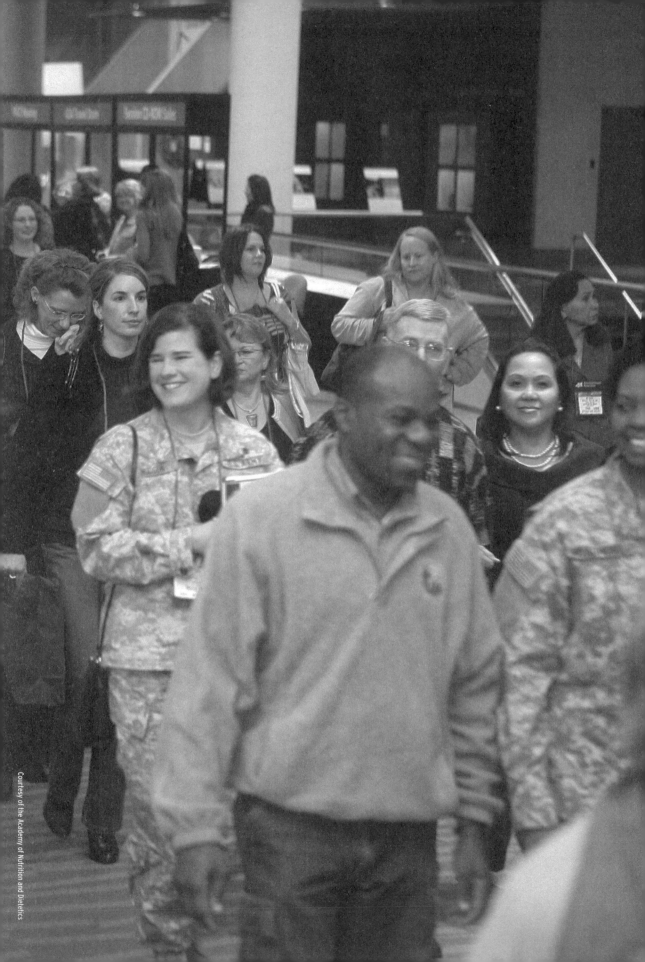

Why Join a Professional Association?

CHAPTER

8

The benefits of membership in a professional association are numerous for those already practicing in the field and for students who aspire to be practicing professionals. Most professional associations offer student membership and provide resources for educational preparation and career building. Specific benefits of student membership include networking with other students in the field; leadership experiences; eligibility for scholarships and awards; access to the latest in online and print media in the field; access to job opportunities; reduced rates at conferences; and special rates on credit cards, car rentals, and hotels.

The Academy of Nutrition and Dietetics

The Academy of Nutrition and Dietetics is the largest association of food and nutrition professionals in the world.[1] Founded in Cleveland, Ohio, in 1917, as the American Dietetic Association, the Academy has grown to more than 100,000 members.[2] The purpose of this chapter is to help you understand the mission, vision, and values of the Academy of Nutrition and Dietetics and to become knowledgeable about its structure and organization. Other professional associations that may be of interest to dietetics professionals are also introduced.

Who Are the Members of the Academy of Nutrition and Dietetics?

The Academy of Nutrition and Dietetics offers five membership classifications: student, active, retired, international, and associate.[3] You may utilize several of these membership categories as you move through your professional life.

The **student member** category is open to anyone who meets one of the following criteria:

- Is a student enrolled in an Accreditation Council for Education in Nutrition and Dietetics (ACEND)-accredited dietetics program or supervised practice program who does not meet requirements for active membership.
- Is a student enrolled in a regionally accredited, postsecondary education program that is non-ACEND accredited (this classification is available to students who state their intent to enter an ACEND-accredited program).
- Is a current active member returning to school on a full-time basis to complete a baccalaureate or advanced degree or to complete an ACEND-accredited supervised practice program (DI or CP). Annual verification is required for this category.

The student membership has a 6-year time limit. The current dues are $50/year.

An **active member** can be any person who has earned the appropriate degree, meets the academic requirements specified by ACEND, and meets one or more of the following criteria:

- Is an RDN or NDTR or has established eligibility to write the registration examination for dietitians or dietetic technicians administered by the Commission on Dietetic Registration (CDR).
- Has completed a baccalaureate degree or a supervised practice program (Plan IV, Plan V, Didactic, DI, CP, AP4, or ISPP programs) accredited or approved by ACEND.
- Is an active member in Dietitians of Canada (DC).
- Has completed an associate degree program for dietetic technicians that ACEND has accredited or approved.
- Has earned a master's or doctoral degree and holds one degree (baccalaureate, master's, or doctoral) in one of the following areas: dietetics, food and nutrition, nutrition, community or public health nutrition, food science, and/or foodservice systems management, or a regionally accredited college or university must confer degrees used to satisfy membership qualifications.

Retired member status can be held by any current active member who is:

- No longer gainfully employed (defined as making equal to or more than the current Federal poverty level for an individual) in dietetic practice or education and is at least 62 years of age.
- Retired on total (permanent) disability.

Academy associate status can be held by anyone who meets the following qualification: has minimum of a bachelor's degree granted by a U.S. regionally accredited college/university or foreign equivalent and training, certification, or license in one of the specified professions. For a list of these professions, see the Academy website at www.eatright.org.

See your dietetics program director for more student member information or call the Academy of Nutrition and Dietetics at 1-800-877-1600.

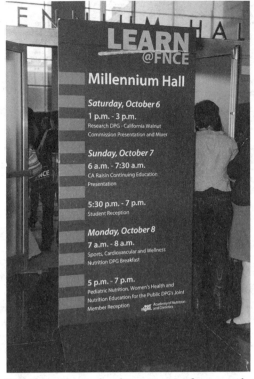

FIGURE 8–1 The Food and Nutrition Conference and Expo (FNCE), the annual meeting of the Academy of Nutrition and Dietetics, offers networking opportunities for students.
Courtesy of the Academy of Nutrition and Dietetics

Alternatively, you can visit the Academy website (www.eatright.org) for membership information. Joining the Academy of Nutrition and Dietetics as a student is an excellent way to learn about the dietetics profession and become familiar with its publications, activities, and other benefits (**Figure 8–1**).

The **international member** category includes any person who:

- Has completed formal training in food, nutrition, or dietetics outside the United States and U.S. territories. Membership in this category requires verification from the country's professional dietetic association or regulatory body.
- Is a student enrolled in food, nutrition, or dietetics educational program outside the United States that is not a U.S. regionally accredited institution and is not accredited by ACEND. This category carries a 6-year limit and is available for international students who state their intent to complete formal training in food, nutrition, or dietetics outside the United States.[4]

Mission, Vision, Philosophy, and Values

In 2008 (when it was still the American Dietetic Association), the Academy of Nutrition and Dietetics Board of Directors endorsed a strategic plan that lays out goals based on the Academy of Nutrition and Dietetics' vision, mission, and values. The plan is reviewed and updated regularly to represent the philosophical base of the Academy.

The vision statement of the Academy of Nutrition and Dietetics "Optimize health through food and nutrition."[5] The Academy's vision statement helps members understand the role the Academy hopes to assume in the future.

The Academy's mission statement is "Empower members to be food and nutrition leaders."[5]

The Academy's values serve as a guide to action and a statement of attributes toward which all dietitians should strive. The Academy's values are:

- Customer focus—meet the needs and exceed the expectations of all customers
- Integrity—act ethically with accountability for lifelong learning and commitment to excellence
- Innovation—embrace change with creativity and strategic thinking
- Social responsibility—make decisions with consideration for inclusivity as well as environmental, economic, and social implications[5]
- Diversity—recognize and respect differences in culture, ethnicity, age, gender, race, creed, religion, sexual orientation, physical ability, politics, and socioeconomic characteristics

Finally, the four strategic goals and outcomes and measures of the Academy of Nutrition and Dietetics that act to guide it in its activities are:

Goal 1: The Public Trusts and Chooses Registered Dietitian Nutritionists as Food, Nutrition, and Health Experts

Outcomes and Measures

- Increases in members' perception of Academy achievement of strategic goals
- Increases in visibility of the Academy to media and consumers, via eatright.org and other media outlets (online, print, and broadcast)
- Maintenance or increases in consumer-rated credibility of RDNs, NDTRs, and the Academy
- Increases in number of RDN and NDTR appointments to external organizations
- Increases in number of invitations to present Academy initiatives to external medical and other healthcare disciplines and their organizations

Goal 2: Academy Members Optimize the Health of Individuals and Populations Served

Outcomes and Measures

- Increases in members' perception of Academy achievement of strategic goals
- Increases in Affiliate Advocacy, Dietetic Practice Group, Academy committee, and Academy Employee Engagement Indices
- Increases in level of collaboration (e.g., more engagement) that strengthen relevant partnerships to promote legislative efforts, including more influential partners, members of Congress, and federal agencies

- Increases in utilization of the Evidence Analysis Library (EAL), an Academy member benefit

Goal 3: Members and Prospective Members View the Academy as Vital to Professional Success

Outcomes and Measures

- Increases in members' perception of Academy achievement of strategic goals
- Increases in Academy membership over time
- Increases in membership market share of nutrition and dietetics practitioners and students in accredited programs
- Increases in perceived value of Academy membership
- Increases in the diversity of nutrition and dietetics professionals
- Increases in utilization of eatrightPRO.org, an Academy member benefit
- Increases in the number of nutrition and dietetics practitioners
- Increases in enrollment in supervised practice programs

Goal 4: Members Collaborate Across Disciplines with International Food and Nutrition Communities

Outcomes and Measures

- Increases in members' perception of Academy achievement of strategic goals
- Increases in number of publications and presentations on international initiatives
- Increases in member engagement in international initiatives
- Increases in number of practice resources for international practitioners in collaboration with international nutrition organizations
- Increases in collaborative research with international colleagues
- Increases in number of professional development opportunities for international practitioners in collaboration with other organizations
- Increases in number of government, World Health Organization (WHO), and United Nations (UN) collaborations

Academy of Nutrition and Dietetics Headquarters

The headquarters of the Academy of Nutrition and Dietetics are located in Chicago, Illinois. It houses the paid staff members who carry on the Academy's day-to-day business. These employees work in assigned groups that serve to support different aspects of the Academy's focus. Also located in the same Chicago location are the Academy of Nutrition and Dietetics Foundation and the offices of the Commission on Dietetic Registration (CDR).

The Foundation funds education initiatives that promote public nutrition, health, and well-being. The Foundation is a nonprofit corporation and is the largest private grantor of scholarships, awards, and research grants in the field of dietetics. This past year, the Foundation awarded more than $1,000,000 to dietetic students and practitioners in the field of dietetics. Students in dietetics and related fields are encouraged to apply for Foundation

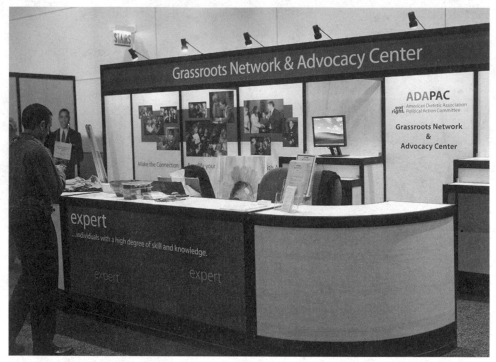

FIGURE 8–2 The ANDPAC (Academy of Nutrition and Dietetics Political Action Committee) booth at the Food and Nutrition Conference and Expo.
Courtesy of the Academy of Nutrition and Dietetics

scholarships. Applications are typically due the middle of February each year, with awards made for the following academic year. Dietetic education program directors receive information about these scholarships every fall.[6]

The CDR is the credentialing arm of the Academy of Nutrition and Dietetics. The CDR credentials individuals who have met its standards for competency to practice in the profession. The function of the CDR is discussed in Chapter 7.[7]

The Academy also retains paid employees at an office in Washington, DC. These employees work on the Academy's behalf on legislative matters that affect the future of the dietetics profession. Members may call the Academy of Nutrition and Dietetics Policy and Advocacy Team in Washington, DC, at 1-800-877-0877 with questions about legislative activities or issues affecting dietetics at the state or federal level (**Figure 8–2**).[8]

The Volunteer Element of the Academy of Nutrition and Dietetics

The officers of the Academy are volunteers who are elected by the membership. Major offices are elected by national ballot; members of particular subgroups, such as Dietetic Practice Groups, elect their own officers.

The work of the Academy is accomplished by two major entities: the Board of Directors and the House of Delegates.

TABLE 8–1

Academy of Nutrition and Dietetics Board of Directors (with Term Length)

Title	Term Length
President	1 year
President-Elect (elected by general membership)	1 year
Past President	1 year
Treasurer	1 year
Treasurer-Elect (elected by general membership)	1 year
Past-Treasurer	1 year
Directors at Large (3, elected by general membership)	3 years
House of Delegates Directors (3, elected by the general membership)	3 years
Speaker	
Speaker-Elect	
Immediate Past-Speaker	
Public Member	3 years
(2, appointed by the Academy Board of Directors for up to a 3-year term)	
Academy Foundation Chair (elected by the Foundation)	1 year
Academy CEO (non-voting)	

Reproduced from the Academy of Nutrition and Dietetics. About the Board of Directors. Available at: http://www.eatrightpro.org/resources/leadership/board-of-directors/about-the-board-of-directors. Accessed February 25, 2016.

The Board of Directors

The Academy of Nutrition and Dietetics is governed by a Board of Directors.[9] To govern the organization, the Academy Board of Directors:

- Sets and monitors strategic direction.
- Oversees fiscal planning.
- Provides leadership for professional initiatives.
- Appoints persons to represent the association.
- Establishes guidelines and policies for appeals, publications, awards, and honors.

The Board of Directors has 19 members (see **Table 8–1**).

The House of Delegates

The Academy of Nutrition and Dietetics House of Delegates (HOD) is the deliberative body of the Academy, acting as the voice of Academy members.[10] The Academy of Nutrition and Dietetics Governing Structure Infographic (**Figure 8–3**) shows the membership, functions, management responsibilities, and frequency of meetings for both the Board of Directors and the HOD.

As shown, the full membership of the HOD meets twice a year, immediately before the start of the Food and Nutrition Conference and Expo each fall (**Figure 8–4**) and at the HOD Mid-Year Meeting; typically held at the end of April or beginning of May. Because delegates are the elected representatives

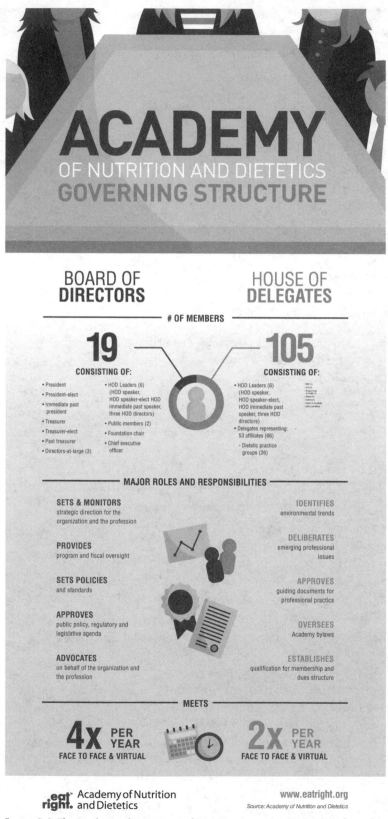

FIGURE 8–3 The Academy of Nutrition and Dietetics Governing Structure Infographic.
Courtesy of the Academy of Nutrition and Dietetics

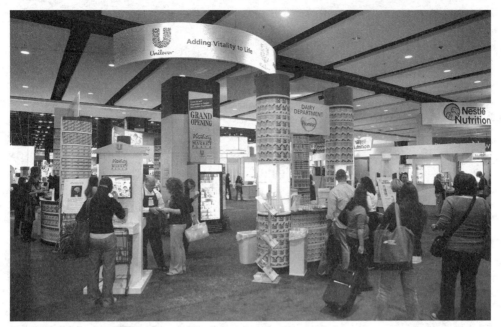

FIGURE 8–4 The exhibit hall at the Food and Nutrition Conference and Expo.
Courtesy of the Academy of Nutrition and Dietetics

of the Academy of Nutrition and Dietetics members in their respective states, they bring to these HOD meetings the views of their constituents back home. Observers are welcome to attend any of these sessions to gain a fuller appreciation of how the work of the Academy is carried out. The formal HOD meeting, during which agenda items are voted on, is held on Sunday each time the HOD meets. It is a formal and impressive event.

State Affiliates and District Dietetic Associations

Each state plus the District of Columbia has its own state dietetic association affiliated with the Academy of Nutrition and Dietetics.

When an individual joins the Academy of Nutrition and Dietetics, a percentage of his or her dues is rebated to the state dietetic association with which he or she wishes to affiliate. Although most individuals are members of the affiliate dietetic association of the state in which they live or work, a 1998 bylaws amendment now allows individuals the option to designate any state dietetic association for their membership. State dietetic associations elect their own officers and host their own meetings once or twice a year.[11]

Each state association is made up of district dietetic associations that serve the needs of dietitians in specific geographic areas within the state. Currently, there are approximately 230 district associations in the United States. District associations may cover a single metropolitan area or several counties. Membership in district associations is not automatic. These groups receive no rebates from the national level and typically charge a separate membership fee to support their programming efforts.

Involvement in district and state dietetic associations is a great way for new dietetics graduates to become involved in a professional organization.

Opportunities for leadership development and personal/professional growth abound in these groups.

Dietetic Practice Groups

Dietetic Practice Groups (DPGs) are composed of individuals who have a common interest in a particular area of dietetics practice, regardless of membership classification or employment status. Anyone with an interest in the particular area of practice can join a DPG, and you can join as many DPGs as desired. A DPG may be formed when at least 300 members petition the House of Delegates Council on Professional Issues to form such a group.

DPGs are national in scope and have their own elected officers and dues. These groups engage in activities that meet the needs of their members, such as producing newsletters or providing continuing education events. They also provide members with the opportunity to develop leadership skills through participation on committees or through appointment or election to offices. The current DPGs of the Academy of Nutrition and Dietetics are listed in **Table 8–2**.[12]

TABLE 8–2

Academy of Nutrition and Dietetics Dietetic Practice Groups

Dietetic Practice Groups	Descriptions
Behavioral Health Nutrition (BHN)	BHN members are the most valued source of food and nutrition services for person with addictions, mental illness, developmental disabilities, and eating disorders.
Clinical Nutrition Management	Managers who direct clinical nutrition programs across the continuum of care.
Diabetes Care and Education (DCE)	Members involved in patient and professional education as well as research for the management of diabetes.
Dietetic Technicians in Practice	Members are advocates for dietetic technicians, registered as dietetic practitioners in providing quality client care.
Dietetics in Health Care Communities	Practitioners typically employed under contract who provide nutrition consultation to acute and long-term care facilities, home care companies, healthcare agencies, and the foodservice industry.
Dietitians in Business and Communications (DBC)	Food and nutrition practitioners who work for or consult with corporations, businesses, and organizations, or who are self-employed or business owners.
Dietitians in Integrative and Functional Medicine	Food and nutrition practitioners who promote the integration of conventional nutrition practices with evidence-based alternatives, including functional and integrative medicine and nutrition genomics.
Dietitians in Nutrition Support (DNS)	Dietitians who integrate the science and practice of enteral and parenteral nutrition in order to provide appropriate nutrition support therapy to individuals encompassing adults, pediatrics, inpatients, outpatients, home care, transplantation, and complex gastrointestinal disorders.
Food and Culinary Professionals	Members who promote food education and culinary skills to enhance quality of life and health of the public.

Healthy Aging	Practitioners who provide and manage nutrition programs and services to older adults in a variety of settings.
Hunger and Environmental Nutrition	Members who lead the future in sustainable and accessible food and water systems through education, research, and action.
Management in Food and Nutrition Systems	Food and nutrition care managers generally employed in healthcare institutions, universities, corrections, and other facilities.
Medical Nutrition Practice Group	Practitioners who practice a wide range of medical nutrition therapy across the continuum of care in a variety of settings.
Nutrition Education for the Public (NEP)	Practitioners involved in the design, implementation, and evaluation of nutrition education programs for target populations.
Nutrition Educators of Health Professionals (NEHP)	Members involved in education and communication with physicians, nurses, dentists, and other healthcare professionals.
Nutrition Entrepreneurs (NE)	NE members shape the future of dietetics practice by pursuing innovative and creative ways of providing nutrition products and services to consumers, industry, media, and business.
Oncology Nutrition	Nutrition professionals involved in the care of cancer patients, cancer prevention, and research.
Pediatric Nutrition	Practitioners who provide nutrition services for the pediatric population in a wide variety of settings.
Public Health/Community Nutrition	Nutrition professionals who work in partnership with healthcare providers, community leaders, and other key stakeholders to serve the public in a variety of roles and settings.
Renal Dietitians	Practitioners who provide medical nutrition services to chronic kidney disease patients in dialysis facilities, clinics, hospitals, university settings, and private practice.
Research	Members who conduct research in various areas to promote practice standards, health policy, and disease prevention.
School Nutrition Services	School foodservice directors, nutrition educators, and corporate dietitians working in the delivery of food service and nutrition education to children.
Sports, Cardiovascular, and Wellness Nutrition	Nutrition practitioners with expertise and skills in promoting the role of nutrition in physical performance, cardiovascular health, wellness, and disordered eating.
Vegetarian Nutrition	Nutrition practitioners who focus on information and resources for plant-based diets.
Weight Management	Practitioners who work in the prevention and treatment of overweight and obesity throughout the life cycle.
Women's Health	Practitioners addressing women's nutrition care issues during the reproductive period through menopause.

Reproduced from Academy of Nutrition and Dietetics. List of Dietetic Practice Groups (DPGs). Available at: http://www.eatrightpro.org/resource/membership/academy-groups/dietetic-practice-groups/list-of-dietetic-practice-groups. Accessed March 3, 2016.

NDEP (Nutrition and Dietetics Educators and Preceptors) is not a DPG but has over 1,100 educator and preceptor members. NDEP's mission is to advocate for and empower educators to lead the profession of nutrition and dietetics. As a result of their mission, the goals of NDEP are: to recognize educators and preceptors as leaders of the profession, support and advance nutrition and dietetic education programs, and support the purposes and goals of The Academy.

In addition to the DPGs, members may also choose to join a Member Interest Group (MIG). MIGs provide a way for members with common interests, issues, or backgrounds to connect. Unlike the affiliate, district, and DPG groups, the MIGs are not based on practice or geographic location. The current MIGs are listed in **Table 8–3**.

TABLE 8–3

Academy of Nutrition and Dietetics Member Interest Groups

MIGs	Descriptions
Asian Indians in Nutrition and Dietetics (AIND)	AIND empowers members to be the leaders in cultural evidence-based practices for people of Indian origin.
Chinese Americans in Dietetics and Nutrition (CADN)	CADN members serve, educate, promote research, and share work experiences within the dietetics and nutrition community to enhance the nutritional status of the Chinese in the United States and worldwide.
Fifty Plus in Nutrition and Dietetics (FPIND)	FPIND focuses on programming, education, careers, and networking targeted at members age 50 years and older.
Filipino Americans in Dietetics and Nutrition (FADAN)	FADAN fosters networking, mentoring, and support for professional issues unique to Filipino-American dietitians, focusing on the diverse culture and ethnicity of this population.
Jewish Member Interest Group (JMIG)	JMIG provides credible resources regarding cultural competencies concerning kosher in observance of kashrut (dietary law) meal service customs to their clients.
Latinos and Hispanics in Dietetics and Nutrition (LAHIDAN)	LAHIDAN fosters the development and improvement of food, nutrition, and health care for Latinos and their families in the United States and related territories.
Muslims in Dietetics and Nutrition (MIDAN)	MIDAN serves members with an interest in cross-cultural awareness and reducing health disparities, specifically as they relate to the Muslim population. This may include those who are of the Muslim faith and/or who work with Muslim clients/patients.
National Organization of Blacks in Dietetics and Nutrition (NOBIDAN)	NOBIDAN provides a forum for professional development of food and nutrition practitioners, while advocating and promoting optimal nutrition and well-being for the general public, particularly those of African-American descent.
National Organization of Men in Nutrition (NOMIN)	NOMIN promotes careers in food and nutrition and professional growth of men through support of research, education, and dissemination of information regarding men's health issues.

| Thirty and Under in Nutrition and Dietetics (TUND) | TUND empowers young practitioners to network and collaborate as the nation's future food and nutrition leaders. |

Reproduced from the Academy of Nutrition and Dietetics. List of Member Interest Groups (MIGs). Available at: http://www.eatrightpro.org/resource/membership/academy-groups/member-interest-groups/member-interest-groups. Accessed March 3, 2016.

Honors and Awards Bestowed by the Academy of Nutrition and Dietetics

Each year, the Academy of Nutrition and Dietetics, the Academy of Nutrition and Dietetics Foundation, and DPGs honor individuals who have demonstrated outstanding contributions to the profession of dietetics. The **Marjorie Hulsizer Copher Award** is the highest honor the Academy can bestow on one of its members. The exemplary career of Marjorie Hulsizer Copher is described in Chapter 1. As the qualifications listed below indicate, the Copher Award honors an Academy member who has been a trailblazer for the profession through active involvement, demonstrated leadership, and professional competence. Qualifications include:

- A member of the Academy.
- Has demonstrated extensive Academy leadership and involvement at national, state, and district levels
- Has recognized professional competence in nutrition and dietetics practice, such as:
  o writing (author, editor, etc.)
  o scientific research
  o management
  o education
  o clinical, community, and/or legislative advocacy
- Has been a source of inspiration to other members to assume leadership roles
- Has been a trailblazer for the profession, such as having created new opportunities for dietitians or technicians
- Has contributed uniquely to the advancement of the profession and/or promoted the Academy's mission, vision, and values
- Has demonstrated devotion to the high standards of the profession

The Copher Award has been presented every year since 1945.[13]

The **Lenna Frances Cooper Memorial Lecture** honors an Academy member who is a role model in the field of nutrition and dietetics and has been recognized as an outstanding speaker. Qualifications include:

- A member of the Academy.
- A recognized speaker:
  o Ability to relate area of expertise to a broad audience
  o Spoken to diverse professional groups within the last 3 to 5 years
  o Reputation as a speaker of note

- Has professional recognition and conduct:
  - Contribution to the profession through service at the national, state, dietetic practice or member interest (DPG/MIG) groups, or district/local levels
  - Unique experiences that are of unusual interest to the profession
  - Source of inspiration and outstanding role model

Topic to be selected by the speaker should be of widespread interest to Academy members and one normally associated with the speaker's work. The presentation of this lecture is a highlight of each Food and Nutrition Conference and Exhibition of the Academy of Nutrition and Dietetics. There has been a Cooper Lecturer recognized every year at the Annual Meeting of the Academy since 1962.[14]

The **Academy of Nutrition and Dietetics Medallion** is awarded each year to honor Academy members who have satisfied the qualifications listed below. Qualifications include the following:

- A member of the Academy for a minimum of 10 years.
- Has contributed to the profession through:
  - exceptional service to the Academy at the national, state, dietetic practice and member interest (DPG/MIG) groups, or district/local levels.
  - exceptional service to other food and nutrition organizations.
  - outstanding professional leadership abilities at all levels of the profession and the community.
  - instrumental in moving the profession forward.
- Has demonstrated characteristics such as:
  - dedication to high standards for the profession.
  - source of inspiration and outstanding role model.
  - promotion of the registered dietitian nutritionist and food and nutrition.
  - service to others in allied fields and the community.

The first Medallions were given in 1976 (**Figure 8–5**), and recipients of this award showcase the diversity of Academy members and their areas of practice.[15]

An **honorary membership** is an award reserved for nonmembers of the Academy who have promoted the Academy's mission, vision, and values using their professional knowledge and expertise. Up to two honorary memberships are given each year to nonmembers based on their professional knowledge, technical expertise and promotion of the Academy's mission, vision and values. The first honorary membership was awarded in 1954.

The **Trailblazer Award** goes to individuals who have demonstrated leadership and advancement of the science at the interface of food science and nutrition/dietetics for at least 5 years.

A reporter, a publication, or a program demonstrative of excellence in nutrition reporting is eligible for the **Media Excellence Award**.

RDNs and NDTRs who have shown innovation, creativity, and leadership in a specific area of practice are candidates for the **Excellence in Practice Awards**.

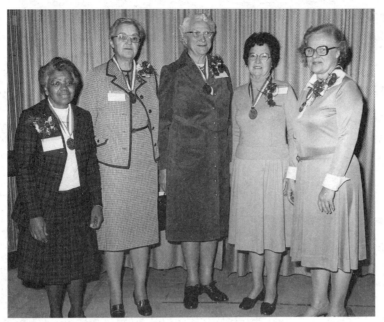

Figure 8–5 The first recipients of the Medallion Award. From left to right: Mildred Bunton, Grace Stumpf, Margaret Terrell, Ruby Linn, and Louise Irwin.
Courtesy of the Academy of Nutrition and Dietetics

The nutrition education of the public, nationally or internationally, by an individual or organization is the focus of the **President's Circle Nutrition Education Award.**

Diversity Awards and Grants include the following:

- Diversity Mini-Grants: $100 to $1,000 grants to support affiliate dietetic associations' outreach to students and professionals from underrepresented groups within the dietetics profession.
- Diversity Promotion Grant: $10,000 grant to support minority recruitment and retention projects by accredited dietetic education programs.
- Diversity Leaders Program: Supports active members from underrepresented groups within the dietetics profession.
- Diversity Action Award: Given to an educational institution, affiliate dietetic association, DPG, or other recognized academy group in recognition of past accomplishments.

The **Academy of Nutrition and Dietetics Foundation Awards and Scholarships** recognize and support dietetics professionals and students. They include the following:

- 17 Continuing Education Awards
- 13 Recognition Awards
- 3 Program Development Awards
- 5 International Awards
- 14 Research Grants totaling $100,000 annually

Foundation Scholarships are awarded annually to deserving students at all levels of study and range from $500 to $10,000.

Affiliate associations may annually select and honor the Recognized Young Dietitian of the Year, Recognized Dietetic Technician of the Year, Emerging Dietetic Leader, and Outstanding Dietitian of the Year awards.

The criteria and selection of the winner for each award are conducted by the affiliate association. Winners' names are listed in the *Journal of the Academy of Nutrition and Dietetics*. Applications for each award can be obtained from each affiliate.

Why Should I Become a Member of the Academy of Nutrition and Dietetics?

Membership in a professional association is a privilege. Professional associations such as the Academy of Nutrition and Dietetics provide opportunities for personal and professional growth, leadership, and lasting friendships. Whereas one dietitian alone may not feel that he or she can make a difference, the strength of more than 100,000 dietitians can make their voices heard in setting public policy or influencing public opinion. The Academy plays a key role in influencing issues such as healthcare reform, food labeling, child nutrition programs, nutrition screening for the elderly, and long-term care. The Academy provides expert testimony at congressional hearings and comments on proposed federal and state legislation. The Academy also publishes position papers, which outline the Academy of Nutrition and Dietetics' stand on a variety of timely, and sometimes controversial, topics. The Academy's website (www.eatright. org) has an extensive listing of member services and benefits.[16] An infographic of the Academy of Nutrition and Dietetics governing structure, previously discussed in this chapter, is shown in Figure 8–3 and infographic of the Academy's organizational units is shown in Figure 8-6. An infographic of the Academy of Nutrition and Dietetics Foundation is shown in **Figure 8–7.**

Other Professional Associations

Dietetics professionals are often involved in numerous professional associations that may relate to their professional activities and interests. Each of these associations has its own mission, agenda, and member benefits. Most of these have a student membership category, which provides an excellent opportunity for students to gain valuable networking experience and resources for professional study and growth (**Table 8–4**).

Summary

Membership in the Academy of Nutrition and Dietetics, your state and district dietetic associations, Academy DPGs, or other professional associations or societies can enhance and enrich your professional and personal growth. Communication, networking, leadership opportunities, and other member benefits are available to those who participate. You determine your own level of involvement and thus your own level of satisfaction. Become actively involved and reap the rewards of an active and involved professional life.

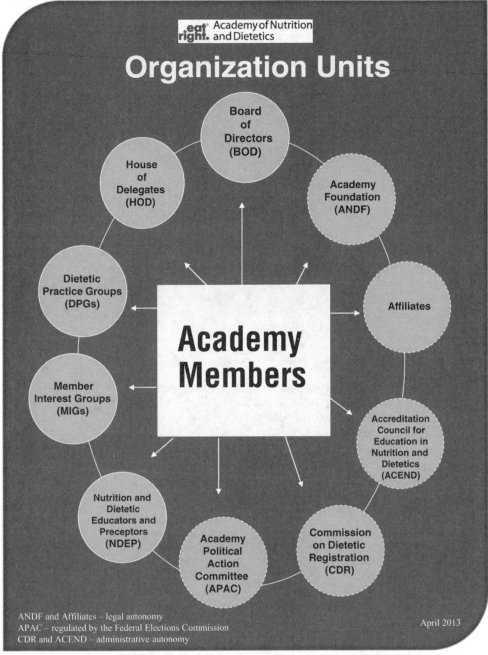

FIGURE 8–6 Academy of Nutrition and Dietetics Organization Units: Academy of Nutrition and Dietetics Foundation and Affiliates—legal autonomy; CDR and ACEND—administrative autonomy; AND-PAC—regulated by the Federal Elections Commission.
Courtesy of the Academy of Nutrition and Dietetics

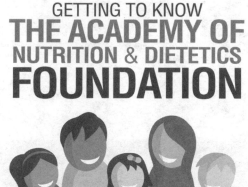

GETTING TO KNOW
THE ACADEMY OF
NUTRITION & DIETETICS
FOUNDATION

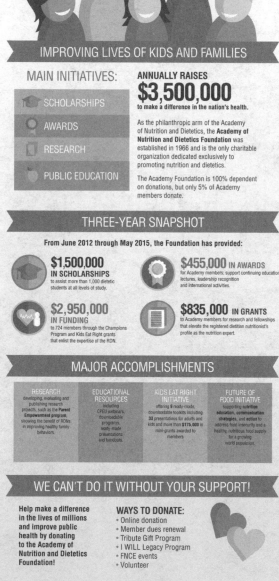

IMPROVING LIVES OF KIDS AND FAMILIES

MAIN INITIATIVES:

- SCHOLARSHIPS
- AWARDS
- RESEARCH
- PUBLIC EDUCATION

ANNUALLY RAISES

$3,500,000
to make a difference in the nation's health.

As the philanthropic arm of the Academy of Nutrition and Dietetics, the **Academy of Nutrition and Dietetics Foundation** was established in 1966 and is the only charitable organization dedicated exclusively to promoting nutrition and dietetics.

The Academy Foundation is 100% dependent on donations, but only 5% of Academy members donate.

THREE-YEAR SNAPSHOT

From June 2012 through May 2015, the Foundation has provided:

$1,500,000 IN SCHOLARSHIPS
to assist more than 1,000 dietetic students at all levels of study.

$455,000 IN AWARDS
for Academy members; support continuing education, lectures, leadership recognition and international activities.

$2,950,000 IN FUNDING
to 724 members through the Champions Program and Kids Eat Right grants that enlist the expertise of the RDN.

$835,000 IN GRANTS
to Academy members for research and fellowships that elevate the registered dietitian nutritionist's profile as the nutrition expert.

MAJOR ACCOMPLISHMENTS

RESEARCH
developing, evaluating and publishing research projects, such as the **Parent Empowerment program**, showing the benefit of RDNs in improving healthy family behaviors.

EDUCATIONAL RESOURCES
including CPEU webinars, downloadable programs, ready-made presentations and handouts.

KIDS EAT RIGHT INITIATIVE
offering 9 ready-made, downloadable toolkits including 33 presentations for adults and kids and more than **$175,000** in mini-grants awarded to members

FUTURE OF FOOD INITIATIVE
supporting **nutrition education, communication strategies,** and action to address food insecurity and a healthy, nutritious food supply for a growing world population.

WE CAN'T DO IT WITHOUT YOUR SUPPORT!

Help make a difference in the lives of millions and improve public health by donating to the Academy of Nutrition and Dietetics Foundation!

WAYS TO DONATE:
- Online donation
- Member dues renewal
- Tribute Gift Program
- I WILL Legacy Program
- FNCE events
- Volunteer

eat right. Academy of Nutrition and Dietetics **Foundation**

www.eatright.org/foundation/donate
SOURCE: The Academy of Nutrition and Dietetics Foundation

FIGURE 8–7 Academy of Nutrition and Dietetics Infographic.
Courtesy of the Academy of Nutrition and Dietetics

TABLE 8–4

Selected Professional Associations

Organization	Address and Phone	Website Address	Publication (s) Available	Student Membership	Membership Dues
American Association of Family and Consumer Sciences (AAFCS)	400 N. Columbus Street, Suite 202, Alexandria, VA 22314 Phone: 703-706-4600	www.aafcs.org	*Journal of Family and Consumer Sciences*	Yes	$50
American College of Sports Medicine (ACSM)	401 W. Michigan Street, Indianapolis, IN 46202-3233 Phone: 317-637-9200	www.acsm.org	*Medicine & Science in Sports & Exercise* *Exercise and Sport Sciences Reviews* *Health & Fitness Journal*	Yes	$10
Academy of Nutrition and Dietetics	120 S. Riverside Plaza, Suite 2000, Chicago, IL 60606-6995 Phone: 800-877-1600	www.eatright.org	*Journal of the Academy of Nutrition and Dietetics* *Food and Nutrition Magazine* *Student Scoop* *Eat Right Weekly*	Yes	$50
American Institute of Wine and Food (AIWF)	26364 Carmel Rancho Lane, Suite 200E, Carmel, CA 93923 Phone: 800-274-2493	www.aiwf.org		No	Regular membership $100
American Public Health Association (APHA)	800 I Street, NW, Washington, DC 20001 Phone: 202-777-2742	www.apha.org	*American Journal of Public Health* *The Nation's Health*	Yes	$75
American Society for Nutrition	9650 Rockville Pike, Bethesda, MD 20814-3998 Phone: 301-634-7050	www.nutrition.org	*The American Journal of Clinical Nutrition* *The Journal of Nutrition*	Yes	$35

(continues)

TABLE 8–4

Selected Professional Associations (Continued)

Organization	Address and Phone	Website Address	Publication (s) Available	Student Membership	Membership Dues
American Society for Parenteral and Enteral Nutrition (ASPEN)	8630 Fenton Street, Suite 412, Silver Spring, MD 20910 Phone: 301-587-2365	www.nutritioncare. org	*Journal of Parenteral and Enteral Nutrition* *Nutrition in Clinical Practice*	Yes	$50
Association for Healthcare Foodservice (AHF)	8400 Westpark Drive, 2nd floor, McLean, VA 22102 Phone: 703-662-0615	www. healthcarefoodservice. org	*Making an Informed Decision* *S.O. Connected*	Yes	Free
Association of Nutrition and Foodservice Professionals	406 Surrey Woods Drive, St. Charles, IL 60174 Phone: 800-323-1908	www.anfponline.org	*Nutrition and Foodservice Edge*	Yes	$64
School Nutrition Association	120 Waterfront Street, Suite 300, National Harbor, MD 20745 Phone: 301-686-3100	https:// schoolnutrition.org	*School Nutrition Magazine* *Journal of Child Nutrition & Management*	Yes	$30
Society for Nutrition Education and Behavior (SNEB)	9100 Purdue Road, Suite 200, Indianapolis, IN 46268 Phone: 800-235-6690	www.sneb.org	*Journal of Nutrition Education & Behavior* *The SNEB eCommunicator*	Yes	$60

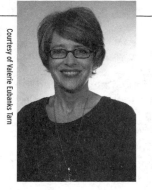

Courtesy of Valerie Eubanks Tarn

Profile of a Professional

Valerie Eubanks Tarn, MS, RDN, LD

Assistant Professor of Pediatrics

Nutrition Faculty and Training Director, Pediatric Pulmonary Center, Division of Pediatric Pulmonary and Sleep Medicine, The University of Alabama at Birmingham, Birmingham, Alabama

Education:

BS in Dietetics, University of Montevallo, Montevallo, Alabama
MS in Clinical Nutrition, The University of Alabama at Birmingham, Birmingham, AL

How did you first hear about dietetics and decide to become a Registered Dietitian?

I shadowed a clinical RD during my freshman year in college, and I soon declared my major in dietetics.

Where did you complete your supervised practice experience?

Dietetic Internship, Emory University, Atlanta, Georgia.

Do you have advanced degree(s)? If so, in what and from where?

- MS in Clinical Nutrition, The University of Alabama at Birmingham
- Pediatric Pulmonary Traineeship, The University of Alabama at Birmingham
- Civitan International Research Center Traineeship, The University of Alabama at Birmingham

How have you been involved professionally?

I have been a leader in my profession through both local and state associations and in the Academy of Nutrition and Dietetics. I currently serve as President for the Birmingham District Dietetic Association and serve on the executive Board with the Alabama Dietetic Association. I have been a member of the Pediatric Nutrition Practice Group for over 20 years and have served as a Mentor, Legislative Chair, Area 3 Coordinator, and Subspecialty Unit Chair. I also serve on various committees at the local, state, and national level related to Maternal and Child Health (MCH).

What honors or awards have you received?

I've received the Recognized Young Dietitian of the Year Award from the State of Alabama and Outstanding Dietitian of the Year from the Birmingham District Dietetic Association.

Briefly describe your career path in dietetics. What are you doing now?

After completing two MCH graduate-level traineeships, I knew my passion was working with children with special healthcare needs. I spent 7 years at Children's Hospital of Alabama as the clinical nutritionist assigned to the pulmonary division. During this time, I discovered a taste for clinical research and spent 10 years working as a research coordinator with the Cystic Fibrosis Research Center. This center includes more than 80 faculty members and has been funded by the National Institutes of Health and Cystic Fibrosis Foundation since 1981. I was the first and only RD employed for this position.

In 2013, I seized an opportunity for career growth as my mentor Nancy Wooldridge, MS, RD, was getting ready to retire after 32 years. Currently, I serve as Nutrition Faculty and Training Director for the Pediatric Pulmonary Center, a (MCH) graduate-level interdisciplinary leadership training program. My main appointment is with University of Alabama at Birmingham as Assistant Professor in Pediatrics in the Division of Pediatric Pulmonary and Sleep Medicine, and I have a secondary appointment as Instructor in the Division of Clinical Nutrition. My academic appointments include didactic and clinical teaching, being a preceptor 10 to 12 months per year to both undergraduate and graduate students, and working with colleagues on research studies.

What excites you about dietetics and the future of our profession?
The opportunities in the field of dietetics continue to grow.

How is teamwork important to you in your position? How have you been involved in team projects?
Building and leading interdisciplinary teams are part of my daily job. Working together as a team collaboratively helps to provide the best patient care to a patient and family. I'm constantly involved in team projects as part of our quality improvement initiative to improve the outcomes of children with special healthcare needs.

What words of wisdom do you have for future dietetics professionals?
Never stop learning. Be exposed to as many opportunities as possible. Find your passion and strive to be a leader who will improve our profession and the health of others.

Suggested Activities

1. Attend a district, state, or national dietetics meeting and share your impressions with your instructor and classmates.
2. Look for the issue of the *Journal of the Academy of Nutrition and Dietetics* that showcases the new officers of the Academy. Read the brief description about each person and find out in what area of dietetics each person works.
3. Are you a student member of the Academy of Nutrition and Dietetics? If so, have you visited the members-only Student Center online at www.eatright.org? What kind of information is found there? If you are not a member, consider joining.
4. Who are the officers of your state dietetic association? What kinds of dietetics positions do they hold? How often does the state association meet?
5. Invite your state's delegate(s) from the Academy's House of Delegates to your class to talk about current issues relevant to dietetics.
6. Which DPGs or MIGs in the Academy of Nutrition and Dietetics are of most interest to you? Visit the website of your top three and look at the membership benefits of each group. How much does it cost to become a member of each group?
7. Does your school have a student nutrition and dietetics club? If so, do you actively participate? If not, attend the next meeting and find out what is going on. If your school does not have a student nutrition and dietetics club, get together with your classmates and form one. Contact other schools that have dietetics programs to find out if they have a nutrition and dietetics club and what types of activities they sponsor.

Selected Websites

- www.eatright.org—The Academy of Nutrition and Dietetics, the world's largest organization of food and nutrition professionals.

References

1. American Dietetic Association. *Promoting Better Health Through Better Nutrition.* Chicago: The American Dietetic Association, 1995.

2. Cassell JA. *Carry the Flame: The History of the American Dietetic Association.* Chicago: The American Dietetic Association, 1990.

3. Academy of Nutrition and Dietetics. Membership Classification Information. Available at: http://www.eatright.org. Accessed November 22, 2015.

4. Academy of Nutrition and Dietetics. Honorary Membership. Available at: http://www.eatright.org. Accessed November 22, 2015.

5. Academy of Nutrition and Dietetics. What Is ADA? Available at: http://www.eatright.org. Accessed November 23, 2015.

6. Academy of Nutrition and Dietetics. ADA Foundation. Available at: http://www.eatright.org. Accessed November 23, 2015.

7. Academy of Nutrition and Dietetics. Commission on Dietetic Registration. Available at: http://www.eatright.org. Accessed November 22, 2015.

8. Academy of Nutrition and Dietetics. Government Affairs. Available at: http://www.eatright.org. Accessed November 23, 2015.

9. Academy of Nutrition and Dietetics. Board of Directors. Available at: http://www.eatright.org. Accessed November 23, 2015.

10. Academy of Nutrition and Dietetics. House of Delegates. Available at: http://www.eatright.org. Accessed November 23, 2015.

11. Academy of Nutrition and Dietetics. Affiliates. Available at: http://www.eatright.org. Accessed November 23, 2015.

12. Academy of Nutrition and Dietetics. Dietetic Practice Groups. Available at: http://www.eatright.org. Accessed November 23, 2015.

13. Academy of Nutrition and Dietetics. Marjorie Hulsizer Copher Award. Available at: http://www.eatright.org. Accessed November 23, 2015.

14. Academy of Nutrition and Dietetics. Lenna Frances Cooper Lecturer. Available at: http://www.eatright.org. Accessed November 23, 2015.

15. Academy of Nutrition and Dietetics. Medallion Award. Available at: http://www.eatright.org. Accessed November 23, 2015.

16. Academy of Nutrition and Dietetics. Member Benefits. Available at: http://www.eatright.org. Accessed November 23, 2015.

PART V

The Future

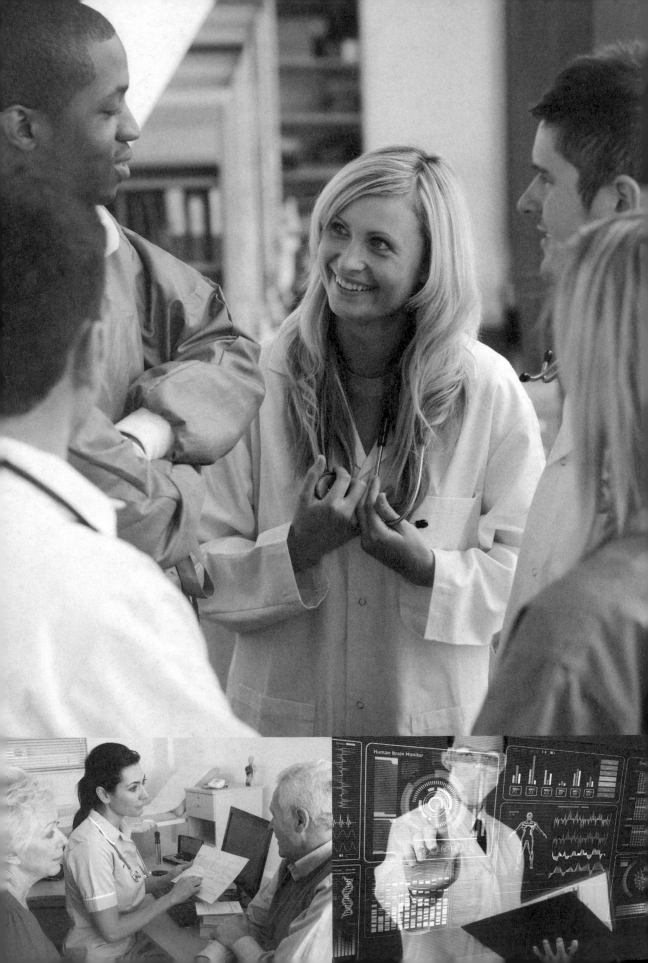

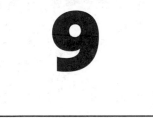

CHAPTER

Trends, Predictions, and Your Future

If we had a crystal ball and could look into the future, what would we see for the future of dietetics? What roles will dietitians play? What areas of practice that are unheard of now will exist in the years ahead? What will be the impact of technology on the practice of dietetics? Will the future needs of our clients be different from what they are today?

The Council on Future Practice (CFP) of the Academy of Nutrition and Dietetics is charged with utilizing a "visioning process" to help visualize the preferred future for the profession of dietetics.[1] The organizational units of the Academy and Academy members provide input to this process to ascertain the change drivers and trends that will affect the future of our profession.

In 2015, the CFP conducted a survey to identify the change drivers and trends, focusing on a 3-year program of work for the Academy (2014–2017).[1] The draft document produced by the CFP and the House of Delegates Leadership Team shares the 10 priority change drivers and their associated trends that are predicted to impact the future of nutrition and dietetics and the Academy over the next 10 to 15 years. The results, reflecting 3,253 total survey responses, are as follows:[1]

"Change Driver: The Approaching Gray Tsunami

- Trend 1: Increasing rates of obesity and chronic diseases among older adults dramatically impact the healthcare system and economic burden of disease.
- Trend 2: Demand for healthcare services is increasing dramatically, although fewer funds are available to cover the cost.
- Trend 3: Disease prevention and health maintenance for the aging population are increasingly the focus to improve quality of life and care and contain costs.
- Trend 4: An aging workforce impacts the economy, businesses, families, and health professions.

Change Driver: Embracing America's Diversity

- Trend 1: Community health workers and other lay educators will continue to be used to reduce health disparities and as a solution to the lack of diversity in the healthcare workforce.
- Trend 2: As the U.S. population grows more diverse, stark differences between what health providers intend to convey in written and oral communications and what patients understand may increase and further exacerbate health disparities.
- Trend 3: Health equality is an increasingly important public health priority because of evolving U.S. racial and ethnic demographics.

Change Driver: Eating to Make the World a Better Place

- Trend 1: Agricultural challenges and rapidly changing technology present entrepreneurial opportunities as food companies seek innovative ways to meet consumer demand for healthy foods and demonstrate their social responsibility.
- Trend 2: Siloed approaches to agriculture, health, sustainability, and economics are being abandoned for transdisciplinary solutions to reduce hunger, poverty, disease, and environmental destruction.
- Trend 3: There is a growing interdependence of countries around the world in sustaining the planet's natural resources.
- Trend 4: Consumers demand increasing levels of food transparency to meet their health, social justice, and environmental stewardship aspirations.

Change Driver: Tailored Health Care to Fit My Genes

- Trend 1: Advances in research and increased demand for personalized health and nutrition result in increased availability and decreased cost of genetic testing.
- Trend 2: Health professionals increasingly manage patient care using genetic profiles, but the science of genetics must continue to advance to inform practice.

Change Driver: The Buck Stops Here

- Trend 1: Healthcare evolutions necessitate increased research and quality improvement activities.
- Trend 2: The application of informatics facilities and optimizes the retrieval, organization, storage, and use of data and information for decision making.
- Trend 3: Practicing RDNs infrequently evaluate and conduct research or access evidence-based resources on a regular basis for guidance in clinical practice.

Change Driver: Making the Healthy Choice the Easy Choice

- Trend 1: Evidence bases and multifactorial interventions that access levels of influence at the environmental, policy, and systems level of the social ecological framework are essential to address population health priorities.
- Trend 2: Institutions, organizations, and governments are increasingly striving for policy changes that are informed by research to help create a culture of health and make healthy choices the easy choices.

- Trend 3: The Affordable Care Act (ACA) paves the way for tremendous growth and unprecedented opportunities in workplace health promotion and disease prevention interventions.
- Trend 4: Hospitals redefine their roles in the continuum of healthcare services and become immersed in the daily culture of the communities they serve.

Change Driver: Creating Collaborative-Ready Health Professionals

- Trend 1: Transdisciplinary professionalism is becoming an essential ideology for a twenty-first century healthcare system.
- Trend 2: Interdisciplinary professional education (IPE) is an increasingly essential strategy for preparing the healthcare workforce for a patient-centered, coordinated, and effective healthcare system.
- Trend 3: A resurgence of interest in IPE has occurred with the goal of team-based care becoming the norm in health care.
- Trend 4: Many difficulties and challenges exist to the successful implementation of IPE, but innovative approaches can help overcome some of the challenges.

Change Driver: Food as Medicine

- Trend 1: Innovations by food and nutrition-related industries are capitalizing on consumers' growing passion for nutrition and health.
- Trend 2: Unprecedented opportunities to lead preventive aspects of health arise from healthcare reform and emerging models of health care.
- Trend 3: Nutrition and medical nutrition therapy (MNT) are poised for prime time with the high prevalence of obesity and its related diseases.

Change Driver: Technological Obsolescence Is Accelerating

- Trend 1: Innovative digital technologies personalize, revolutionize, and increase access to health care.
- Trend 2: Technological applications, economics, and student demands disrupt traditional educational institutions.
- Trend 3: Technological advances impact work settings and change how, when, and where people work.
- Trend 4: The digital age is transforming the next-generation food system.

Change Driver: Simulations Stimulate Strong Skills

- Trend 1: Simulations help address increased complexity of health care, higher patient acuity levels, and patient safety.
- Trend 2: Accountability of care, pay-for-performance, and financial penalties for provider errors spur interest in simulations.
- Trend 3: The use of simulations increases in response to cost cutting in higher education and reduction in the availability of clinical placements for students.
- Trend 4: The desire to improve critical thinking skills of learners drives the development and use of simulations."[1]

Implications for Dietetics Practice

Although trends are interesting to explore, this doesn't mean they will necessarily materialize. No one has yet discovered how to predict the future! However, the systematic forecast of trends and patterns by futurists is critical to planning—whether for a professional organization or for one's personal future. Following are a few of the implications of these change drivers and trends on dietetics practice and your future as an RDN or NDTR.

- There will be an increased demand for home-based and community-based food and nutrition services as more and more seniors opt to stay in their own homes as long as possible to avoid the move to costly long-term care facilities. This will necessitate more in-depth training in geriatric nutrition and geriatric specialties for RDNs and NDTRs. And, as older RDNs and NDTRs retire, we must ensure an adequate supply of new practitioners to take their places.[2,3]

- RDNs and NDTRs must be culturally competent to be able to interact effectively and appropriately with our country's increasingly diverse population. We must figure out ways to recruit and retain dietetic students from minority and underrepresented groups to be the dietetics professionals of the future. Future RDNs and NDTRs need to increase their language skills, particularly working to enhance their fluency in languages such as Spanish, French, Arabic, and Cantonese. More research is needed to collect and analyze data to track and address disparities in health outcomes in racial and ethnic groups.[1]

- Future dietetics professionals need to be leaders in the realm of the interrelationship between diet, health, and the environment as the public's interest in this area is higher than ever before. Understanding organics, local foods, issues of food sustainability, food and water conservation, and how the food chain and food sector of our economy works will be vital for RDNs and NDTRs to step up to positions of leadership.

- Genetic testing so that individuals can learn about their own risk for chronic disease is inevitable. Information gained from such testing can help RDNs plan individual, specific nutrition interventions. Prospective RDNs who wish to work in this arena should prepare for advanced study and practice in the area of genetics, genetic testing, and nutrigenomics and for working closely with interdisciplinary team members.

- Future dietetics professionals must understand and apply research to their practice. It is also critical to understand costs of nutrition intervention and whether these interventions are cost effective and lead to improved outcomes. RDNs and NDTRs must understand that every action has cost implications and be ready to demonstrate their worth to the client and to the organization for which they work. RDNs must be prepared to provide outcomes data to support their interventions.

- Future RDNs and NDTRs must prepare themselves for emerging areas of dietetics practice, particularly in community settings. Becoming engaged in advocacy and public policy is critical. Workplace health promotion is going to grow in importance, and dietetics professionals can be key players in this important area.

- Dietetics education must become more collaborative with other health-care professions and consider including interdisciplinary professional education competencies for certification and licensure. Dietetics programs need to increase opportunities for dietetic students to collaborate with and learn from other health professions students because this will enable all future healthcare professionals to better understand the roles played by each.
- RDNs and NDTRs should position themselves for emerging jobs in the food industry, particularly as restaurants and vending machine companies work to meet the ACA mandates for nutrition labeling. Health promotion and disease prevention will become a competitive marketplace, and dietetics entrepreneurs need to be prepared to seize opportunities in this arena.
- As technology advances at warp speed, dietetics professionals need to be ready to become involved in development of expert systems, mobile app research and development, and other technological innovations. Digital literacy must be a part of dietetics education to prepare graduates for digital healthcare technologies of the future. RDNs should be knowledgeable about informatics and data management.
- Simulation needs to become an important part of dietetics education and integrated into dietetics curricula. Development of high-quality simulations can be expensive and time consuming but can reap huge benefits in preparing students for practice, particularly as clinical sites become more and more scarce.

The Future for Dietetics Professionals

According to the Bureau of Labor Statistics of the U.S. Department of Labor, the job market for dietetics professionals continues to grow, with a projected growth rate of 16% from 2014 to 2024, a much greater growth rate than the average for all occupations.[4] According to the Department of Labor, job growth will result from an increasing emphasis on disease prevention through improved dietary habits. A growing and aging population will boost demand for nutritional counseling and treatment in hospitals, residential care facilities, schools, prisons, community health programs, and home healthcare agencies. Public interest in nutrition and increased emphasis on health education and prudent lifestyles will also spur demand, especially in foodservice management. Entrepreneurs such as personal chefs and trainers who prepare and cook food for clients in their homes and give personal nutrition advice are challenging dietetics professionals. Some dietitians are seeking additional credentials, such as those discussed in Chapter 7, to broaden the services they are able to deliver. Dietitians are also gaining new knowledge and skills in disciplines such as pharmacy, exercise physiology, biochemistry, culinary arts, communication, business, and other areas.

Summary

The future of dietetics is dynamic and exciting. Entrepreneurial dietitians, who see change as opportunity, will be the ones who take dietetics through the next century. Dietitians must be willing to seize opportunities to market themselves and their abilities in new and exciting ways. If we are to fulfill the Academy's vision to optimize the nation's health through food and nutrition and the Academy's mission to empower members to be the nation's food and nutrition leaders,[5] we must look to the future with energy, enthusiasm, and an entrepreneurial spirit. The profession of dietetics has a bright and exciting future. Only your energy level and imagination will limit you. Prepare now to be a part of that bright future!

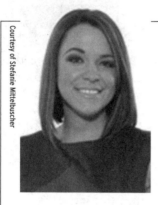

Courtesy of Stefanie Mittelbuscher

Profile of a Professional

Stefanie Mittelbuscher, DTR

Patient Services Manager
St. Mary's Health Center, St. Louis, Missouri

Education:
AAS in Dietetics, St. Louis Community College, St. Louis, Missouri
BS in Accounting, University of Missouri–St. Louis, St. Louis, Missouri

How did you first hear about dietetics and decide to become a Dietetic Technician, Registered?
My mother is a dietitian, so I have had an interest in food since a young age. While trying to decide what major to enroll in, she suggested I check out a dietetic technician program. After that, I knew it was what I wanted to do.

In what types of facilities did you gain your supervised practice experience?
My first practicum was at a small regional hospital in foodservice management. This allowed me to see the big picture of an operation and got me even more excited for my future career path. I was able to assist with inventory, ordering, and even supervision of staff. After my practicum, they hired me as a p.r.n. (as needed) dietary worker, which allowed me to gain more experience.

My second practicum was at a large hospital in clinical nutrition. I was able to do assessments, order supplements, obtain diet histories, and give diet instruction. Although this wasn't my emphasis area, it did give me a well-rounded view of how the foodservice and clinical nutrition operations impact each other.

My last practicum was through a local school district. I was able to spend time in meal preparation and planning for several high schools, elementary schools, and middle schools. This allowed me to explore an area of dietetics that I honestly hadn't thought much about previously, but now I see has a larger impact on the overall nutrition and health of our population.

Do you have an advanced degree?
No, not at this point. I just recently received my Bachelor of Science degree in accounting from the University of Missouri–St. Louis. I always knew I wanted to go back to school, but I felt that pursuing the RD credential was not the right path for me. I know that foodservice management is my field, and I felt that while the RD would give me more science knowledge, I didn't feel it would help me further my management career. The DTR program gave me a solid base in nutrition that allows me to perform at a high level at my current position. A business degree seemed more logical to help me further my career path. Additionally, accounting gave me an area of specialty that adds to my professional skills.

How have you been involved professionally?
I served as the DTR representative for the Commission on Dietetic Registration (CDR) of the Academy of Nutrition and Dietetics from 2012 to 2015. During this time,

I worked on both the Appeals Panel and the Exam Panel. I also spent 1 year as chair of the Appeals Panel.

What honors or awards have you received?
During my time at Florissant Valley Community College, I was awarded Outstanding Dietetics Student–Food Service Management. Additionally, in 2013, I was recognized as the Outstanding Dietetic Technician for the state of Missouri.

Briefly describe your career path in dietetics. What are you doing now?
I like to think my career path in dietetics started before I was even officially "in" dietetics. My first job was as a hostess at a restaurant. This was really my first "management" experience, as the hostess manages the whole flow of the restaurant for the customers and the workers. From there, I entered the DTR program and graduated in 2005.

My first job as a DTR was at a small children's orthopedic hospital called Shriners Hospital for Children. This allowed me to work both in clinical nutrition and foodservice management and further solidified my passion for management.

A short time later I accepted a position with Sodexo contract management company to work as a patient services manager for a local hospital that was struggling after implementing the room service approach for delivering food to their patients. I was able to successfully improve the operational efficiency as well as the patient satisfaction scores. That brings me to where I am today. I received a promotion with Sodexo to move to another hospital within the same system and do much the same; I help the operational efficiency of room service and, in turn, improve patient satisfaction.

What excites you about dietetics and the future of our profession?
The future of our profession is an open book, and we have the power to make it what we want. Academy of Nutrition and Dietetics members need to get involved with issues they are passionate about, and we need more members to advocate for the profession and the many avenues we can impact. I think our profession has such a large influence on the health of the nation and has the power to change many of the epidemics in our world. I have recently become interested in school nutrition as I see this is the forefront of nutrition change for our country.

How is teamwork important to you in your position? How have you been involved in team projects?
Teamwork is the base of any action within my position. I have to promote teamwork among my employees in order to have an efficient operation. Teamwork also allows them to have a more satisfying work environment, which, in turn, causes them to help satisfy our patients. I have been involved in many team projects and I have found over and again that the main thing that makes a team work is COMMUNICATION!

What words of wisdom do you have for future professionals?
Dream big! The profession is in your hands. Get involved and work toward goals for our profession that you are passionate about!

Suggested Activities

1. Review copies of the *Journal of the Academy of Nutrition and Dietetics* and the Academy's *Food & Nutrition* magazine for the past year. What hot topics are being discussed in these publications? How much do you know about these topics? How do you think these topics may affect your future practice in dietetics?

2. Read current issues of popular newspapers or newsmagazines, such as *The Wall Street Journal, Time, Newsweek,* and so on. Look specifically for articles that might relate to dietetic practice, including topics related to health, food, nutrition, foodservice, public health, and others. What implications might these topics have for dietetics?

3. Review the "President's Page" in each issue of the *Journal of the Academy of Nutrition and Dietetics.* What topics have been discussed? What issues are facing the profession of dietetics or the Academy of Nutrition and Dietetics?

4. Search online for the websites of some entrepreneurial dietitians and see what kinds of services they provide. Some websites of entrepreneurial dietitians are provided in the following "Selected Websites" section.

Selected Websites

- www.nancyclarkrd.com—Nancy Clark, MS, RD, CSSD, is an internationally known sports nutritionist and best-selling author trusted by many top athletes.
- www.nutritionexpert.com—Mitzi Dulan, RD, CSSD, is a nutrition and health spokesperson, author, and speaker.
- http://www.healthykidschallenge.com—Healthy Kids Challenge is a nationally recognized 501(c)3 nonprofit led by registered licensed dietitians with years of school, program, and community wellness experience.
- http://foodfitfabulous.com—Susan Mitchell, PhD, RDN, LDN, FADA, is a nutrition spokesperson, consultant, and author/freelance writer. Regina Ragone, MS, RDN, is Food Director for *Family Circle* magazine, blogger, and author.
- http://ellynsatterinstitute.org—Ellyn Satter, MS, RDN, MSSW, at the Ellyn Satter Institute provides resources for professionals and the public in the area of eating and feeding.
- http://nutritionforkids.com/24_Carrot.htm—Connie Evers, MS, RDN, CSSD, founded 24 Carrot Press, which publishes titles that promote the nutritional health of children and adolescents.

References

1. Academy of Nutrition and Dietetics, Council on Future Practice, Visioning Process Workgroup, Kicklighter J, Dorner B, Hunter AM, Kyle M, Prescott M, Roberts S, Spear B. Change drivers and trends driving the profession: A prelude to the visioning report 2017. Available at: http://www.eatrightpro.org/resource/leadership/volunteering/committee-leader-resources/visioning-process. Published November 12, 2015. Accessed January 16, 2016.

2. Academy of Nutrition and Dietetics. *Academy of Nutrition and Dietetics Compensation and Benefits Survey of the Dietetics Profession 2013.* Chicago: Academy of Nutrition and Dietetics; 2013.

3. Accreditation Council for Education in Nutrition and Dietetics. Rationale for Future Education Preparation of Nutrition and Dietetics Practitioners. ACEND Website. Available at: www.eatrightacend.org/ACEND/content.aspx?id=6442485290. Published February 2015. Updated August 2015. Accessed January 15, 2016.

4. U.S. Bureau of Labor Statistics. Occupational Outlook Handbook: Dietitians and Nutritionists. Available at: http://www.bls.gov/ooh/healthcare/dietitians-and-nutritionists.htm. Accessed January 15, 2016.

5. Academy of Nutrition and Dietetics. Academy Mission and Vision. Available at: http://www.eatrightpro.org/resources/about-us/academy-vision-and-mission. Accessed January 15, 2016.

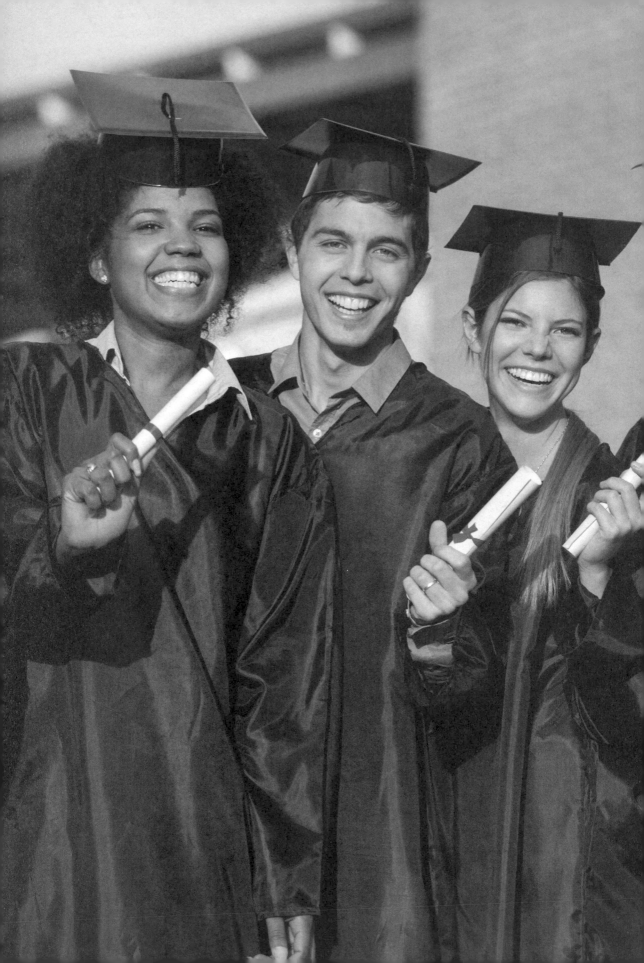

Crossing the Bridge: From Student to Professional

Are you ready for the real world? When you arrived on campus as a freshman, your goal may have been survival—academic and social. With the voluminous amount of reading and writing required by your classes, seemingly endless time spent in labs, juggling the demands of work and school, and fitting in some extracurricular activities, very little time is left to think about the next step—until senior year, when reality hits! What's next—graduate school, work, internship, marriage, family, travel, money? Where, when, and how decisions abound. This can be a very stressful time, not only because of the important decisions that must be made, but also because of the changes that must be faced. What will be the same and what will be different when you leave college to enter your profession? How difficult will it be to cross that bridge? And how can you make the transition successfully?

Transitions, in general, are challenging periods of one's life, whether it is elementary to middle school, high school to college, undergraduate to graduate school, graduate school to a professional life, reentering the professional world after taking time off, or changing career paths. This chapter focuses on the transition from school to profession, with the realization that it may be somewhat different in every case. For some, it may be more challenging than for others. For most, however, some strategies to manage the stresses associated with the changes that are faced can lay the foundation for career success. Engaging in self-assessment and developing clearly defined career goals, as discussed in Chapter 4, compose the first step.

How does the student role differ from the professional role? If you are reading this text, you are already familiar with the student role. So, what does it mean to be a professional? Consider someone whom you would describe as professional. If you were asked to describe this person, what would you say? Would you say that he or she is knowledgeable, ethical, caring, well dressed and well groomed, competent, assertive, responsible, committed to work and profession, a team player, and respectful of others? In this chapter, we examine the conduct, aims, and qualities considered characteristic of the dietetics profession. We emphasize the importance of showing respect and concern for people, being knowledgeable and keeping current with the latest research in one's area of practice, adhering to the strictest ethical standards, and having a commitment to the profession.

Professional Advice

The consistent piece of advice from those who have been there is that you need to figure out how to make the transition from student to professional while you are still in school, and the earlier the better. "Figuring it out" includes defining your career goals, making a commitment to manage your future, identifying a mentor, utilizing networking opportunities, and taking some risks.

Self-assessment and determining career goals are discussed in Chapter 4, "Beginning Your Path to Success in Dietetics." With some definite, possible, tentative, or interesting career goals in mind, the next step is to decide which internships, graduate programs, or companies and jobs can help you to achieve these goals. Research possibilities early in your college career to determine what knowledge, skills, work experience, and other qualities will make you a good candidate for your choices. This information will be helpful in making decisions on elective courses, fieldwork experiences, part-time jobs, extracurricular activities, service learning, and volunteer opportunities.

Seeking out professional advice should also occur early in your college career. The obvious way to seek professional advice is to talk to professionals. As a student, you have the opportunity to talk to professors in the field. Some students are reluctant to approach professors and instead wait for them to offer help. This is one time that it may be necessary to take the initiative. Professors are busy people, too, juggling departmental, professional, and personal demands on their time. But most faculty members want to help students in their program. You simply have to ask.

Interviewing dietetic practitioners who work in the areas of practice in which you are interested may also be helpful. In addition to taking the initiative to create some informal interactions with professors and other professionals, it is a good idea to take advantage of the student memberships offered by most professional associations. The printed materials that are sent to members can give you a good overview of the field, issues faced by the profession, current job listings, research being conducted, and calendars of professional events that provide networking and professional development opportunities.

Developing a relationship with a professional of a more formal nature, a mentor, can provide invaluable help during the transition as well as during the early stages of a career transition. A **mentor** is a wise and trusted counselor and guide. Mentoring is a special kind of caring, supportive relationship or partnership between two people based on trust and respect. Mentors share their knowledge and experience with mentees (protégés) to help them define and reach their goals. Faculty members and preceptors often serve as early mentors to students (**Figure 10–1**).

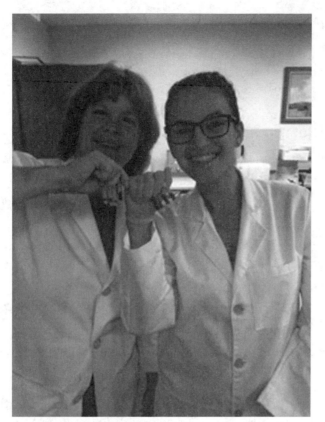

Figure 10–1 An intern and her clinical preceptor meet.
Courtesy of Susan Helm, PhD, RDN, Pepperdine University

According to the late Pauline Schatz, EdD, RD, a longtime proponent of mentoring:

Positive relationships benefit the mentor, mentee, and society. In a nurturing relationship the mentor finds gratification providing guidance for the mentee to reach his/her goals. The mentee meets with a role model who motivates and guides the mentee toward the fulfillment of possibilities and personal goals. By practicing in a safe, stable environment, the mentee gains confidence while developing new skills. Both mentor and mentee are able to assess their knowledge and experience as well as take advantage of the opportunity for self-reflection. This results in a higher level of productivity. Society benefits not only from the increased productivity but also in this relationship the mentor, through the mentee, is often able to develop a legacy for future leadership that in turn will provide guidance for a new generation.[1]

Although mentoring has been traditionally a one-on-one relationship, the team approach can be applied here as well. "Talent teams" have been formed to offer professional advice, to help solve problems, and to provide opportunities for collaboration or referrals, stimulation, and encouragement. A talent team is essentially organized lateral mentoring. Just like traditional mentoring, it involves a commitment to sharing time and information. The difference is that everyone is on the same level, and all ideas and feedback are of equal importance and consideration. Such a team may include a nutrition educator, a behavior change consultant, a national healthcare consultant, a communications consultant, a product development manager, and a marketing and research consultant.[2]

You Are Entering a Helping Profession

By its very nature, dietetics is a helping profession. Dietetic practice involves service. The way this service is delivered is critically important. Respect, caring, and concern for people and their value systems are basic to the concept of professionalism. These characteristics may be manifested in many ways, not the least of which is respect for the dignity of each and every person. An understanding of individual differences, such as gender, ethnicity, and religion, is also critical for effective practice.

Lifelong Learning and Professional Development

One of the requirements of professional practice is the maintenance of competence. Each practitioner is responsible for devising and implementing professional development strategies. The Academy of Nutrition and Dietetics' Center for Professional Development offers many opportunities for students and practitioners to stay up-to-date in food and nutrition, build knowledge, and enhance skills, which, in turn, will help with career advancement (**Figure 10–2**).

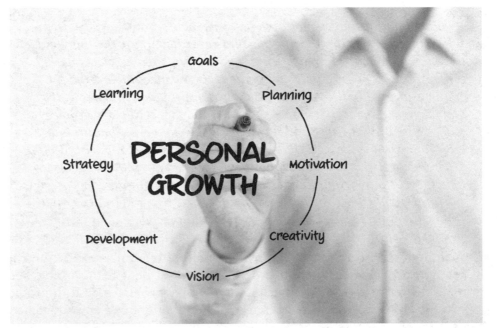

FIGURE 10–2 Personal growth diagram.
© Bloomua/Shutterstock

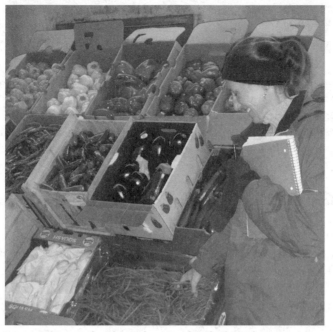

FIGURE 10–3 A student learns how to select fresh produce on a trip to the wholesale market.
Courtesy of Lari Bright

The rapidly changing character and increasing complexity of dietetics practice demands continual updating of the practitioner's knowledge, skills, and understanding. Professional development recognizes an individual's investment of time and effort required for exemplary professional performance throughout a career. Personal professional development is the lifelong process of active participation in learning activities that assist in maintaining and advancing continuing competence in professional practice. Professional development begins within the entry-level educational program and continues throughout the career of the dietetics professional (**Figure 10–3**).[3]

The Academy's strategic plan identifies lifelong learning as one of the values on which the future of dietetics will be built. The role of the CDR and the Professional Development Portfolio in ensuring practitioner competence were discussed in Chapters 4, 5, and 7.

Standards of Professional Practice

The phrases "Standards of Practice (SOP)" and "Standards of Professional Performance(SOPP),"[4] as used by the Academy, refer to a set of defined statements of a dietetic professional's responsibility for providing services, regardless of the setting, project, case, or situation. They may be used by credentialed practitioners for self-evaluation and to determine the education and skills needed to advance their own level of practice. There are also SOP and SOPP standards for areas of focus, such as diabetes, health promotion in higher education, nutrition in athletic performance, diagnosis and management of food allergy, and nutrition informatics.

Professional Ethics

Ethical issues[5] faced by members of the dietetics profession are as diverse as the settings in which members practice. In medical and clinical settings, patients' rights, confidentiality of information, and the provision of food and water are the primary issues that must be confronted. In foodservice settings, ethical issues revolve around the management of money, personnel, materials, and time. In research and education, issues of plagiarism and research designs involving animals or human beings are issues of ethical concern.

Every professional association must address the issue of acceptable professional behavior. This is usually accomplished through a written document called a code of ethics. The code describes the philosophy and expectations of conduct to which the association agrees its members should adhere. The Code of Ethics for the Profession of Dietetics can be found on the Academy of Nutrition and Dietetics' website (www.eatright.org) and is discussed in Chapter 7. The Code of Ethics is voluntary and enforceable. It challenges all members, RDNs, and NDTRs to uphold ethical principles, and it establishes a fair system to deal with complaints about members and credentialed practitioners from peers and the public.

The purpose of a professional code of ethics is to reflect the principles of the profession and to provide an outline of the obligations of the member of that profession to self, client, society, and the profession. The Code of Ethics for the Profession of Dietetics addresses the provision of professional services, the accurate presentation of credentials and qualifications, standards for avoiding conflict of interest, and accountability for professional competence in practice. The Code also speaks to compliance with laws and regulations concerning the profession; presentation of substantiated information; confidentiality of information; the honesty, integrity, and fairness of the member; and the obligation to uphold the standards of the profession by reporting apparent violations.

New members joining the Academy receive a copy of the Code of Ethics and sign a statement stating that they will abide by it. The review process for violations of this code includes a review of the complaint, an investigation, a hearing, and, finally, a decision and recommendation. The respondent may be acquitted or, if found guilty, censored, temporarily suspended, or expelled from membership.

Commitment to the Profession

Those demonstrating professionalism in dietetic practice have a sense of commitment to the growth of the profession, both as a field of intellectual endeavor and as a society in which people of similar purposes band together. This commitment is best demonstrated by active participation in a professional association. Professional associations rely heavily on the work of volunteers at all levels—local, state, and national. Through this collective energy of many professionals working together, an association becomes dynamic and productive. As Peter Drucker said, "No organization can do better than the people it has."[6]

The benefits of professional association membership are both tangible and intangible. The tangible benefits may include receipt of publications, continuing education opportunities, lobbying on key legislative issues, public relations and marketing efforts, public recognition of professional achievements, student scholarship programs, member loan programs, discounts on rental cars and publications, travel programs, association-sponsored credit cards, group-rate medical and life insurance, and professional liability insurance— to mention a few.

Of even greater importance are the intangible benefits that accrue from professional association involvement. The friendships that develop, the opportunity to hone leadership skills, the sense of creative stimulation, the excitement of being a part of the action, and the opportunity to impact issues and shape policy for the good of the profession are good reasons to volunteer at some level of commitment (**Figure 10–4**).

For students, there are additional advantages of active participation. Students have an opportunity to:

- Develop skills in public speaking, writing, and program planning and organizing.
- Network with dietitians, technicians, and other students.
- Observe professional role models.
- Enhance visibility for scholarships, internships, and future employment.

The biggest drawback of active involvement in a professional association is the time commitment required. Frustrations may also arise when costs exceed the resources available for certain plans or when members disagree. But these are minor considerations when one considers the risk of not being involved.

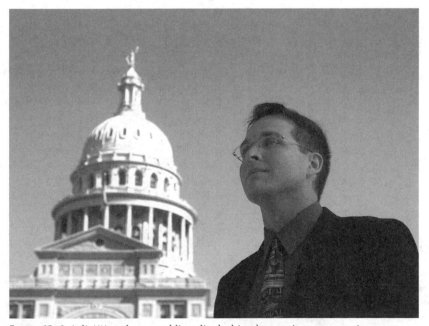

FIGURE 10–4 A dietitian shapes public policy by his advocacy in government.
© David Gilder/Shutterstock

Finally, Some Tips for Career Success

"Whatever the struggle,
Continue to climb,
For it may only be
One more step to your success!"

The Pyramid of Success, shown in **Figure 10–5,** was developed by legendary basketball Coach John Wooden. It took him hundreds of hours of reflection and 14 years of hard work to develop. The boxes on the pyramid comprise the characteristics that Coach Wooden believed essential for success in any and all endeavors. They include:

- *Competitive greatness:* Enjoy the difficult challenges.
- *Poise:* Be at ease in any situation; don't fight yourself.
- *Confidence:* Be prepared and keep things in their proper perspective.
- *Condition:* Mental, moral, and physical condition; rest, exercise, and diet must be considered, moderation must be practiced, and dissipation must be eliminated.
- *Skill:* Knowledge of and the ability to properly and quickly execute the fundamentals; be prepared, and cover every little detail.
- *Team spirit:* A genuine consideration for others, an eagerness to sacrifice personal interest of glory for the welfare of all.
- *Self-control:* Keep emotions under control; good judgment and common sense are essential.
- *Alertness:* Observe constantly; be eager to learn.
- *Initiative:* Cultivate the ability to make decisions and think alone; do not be afraid of failure but learn from it.

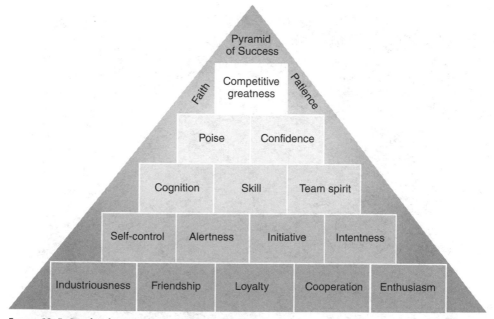

FIGURE 10–5 Coach John Wooden's Pyramid of Success.

Reproduced from Wooden : A lifetime of observations and reflections on and off the court by WOODEN, JOHN R.; JAMISON, STEVE © 1997 Reproduced with permission of MCGRAW-HILL COMPANIES, INC.

- *Intentness:* Set realistic goals; concentrate by resisting all temptations and being determined and persistent.
- *Industriousness:* Worthwhile results come from hard work and careful planning.
- *Friendship:* Requires mutual esteem, respect, and devotion; like marriage, it must not be taken for granted but requires a joint effort.
- *Loyalty:* Keep your self-respect.
- *Cooperation:* Listen if you want to be heard; be interested in finding the best way, not in having your own way.
- *Enthusiasm:* Truly enjoy what you are doing.[7]

Wooden also recommends the development of the following 10 qualities for success:

1. Faith, through prayer
2. Patience, good things take time
3. Fight, determined effort
4. Integrity, purity of intention
5. Resourcefulness, proper judgment
6. Reliability, creates respect
7. Adaptability, to any situation
8. Honesty, in thought and action
9. Ambition, for noble goals
10. Sincerity, keeps friends[7]

High self-esteem and open-mindedness are embedded in several areas of the triangle. A positive attitude is a trait that successful practitioners share. Many of these traits are developed, not inborn. As Abraham Lincoln said, "Most of us are about as happy as we make up our minds to be." A positive outlook can be developed in a number of ways. Dr. Wolf Rinke, in his books *Positive Attitude: The Key to Peak Performance* (2003) and *The 6 Success Strategies for Winning at Life, Love, and Business* (1996), offers a number of suggestions, including:

- Build a network of positive colleagues—associate with positive people.
- Reformulate your language by using positive words rather than negative.
- When anyone asks, "How are you doing?" answer "GREAT!" with enthusiasm.
- Appreciate yourself for who you are rather than who you think you ought to be.
- Love people for the way they are not for the way you think they ought to be.
- Make it a habit to treat every person you meet as if he or she were the most important person in the world.
- Live in the present—let go of the past.
- Accept that mistakes are part of life, and learn from them.
- In teamwork, do more than is expected of you.
- Spend less time watching television unless it is purposeful and positive programming.

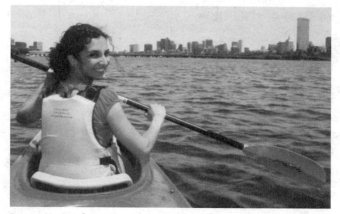

Figure 10–6 A dietitian enjoys an afternoon canoeing on the Charles River.
Courtesy of Michele Coelho, RD

- Spend the newly found time doing something that will enrich you—reading, a new hobby, professional development activities, and so on.
- Use "I" statements, as described in Chapter 3.
- Say good things about people or say nothing at all.
- Smile often[8–10] (**Figure 10–6**).

Summary

Crossing the bridge from student to professional can be a smooth journey if plans are made early and carefully. Knowing who you are and where you want to go, seeking the advice and mentorship of others, and taking advantage of networking opportunities are some of the ways to make the change less stressful. An internship, graduate school, a practicum, a traineeship, and supervised fieldwork all are helpful ways of bridging the differences between the classroom and the profession.

The profession of dietetics has been shaped and molded by dynamic and dedicated individuals whose careers have made a difference. The profession requires a team approach, with each member of the team being the very embodiment of professionalism—knowledgeable, caring, concerned, respectful, ethical, committed to the profession, and active in the professional organization. The dietetic team member has an essential orientation to the interest of others—the patient, the client, and the community. The dietetic team member is unquestionably ethical in all matters. He or she is committed to preserving the credibility and dignity of the profession and believes that the practice of dietetics has an impact on the quality of life of others. Putting aside personal benefits and/or costs, the dietetic team member recognizes the importance of professional association involvement for the good of the profession as a whole.

Making a smooth transition from school to profession puts you on the road to career success. Know yourself, manage yourself, and motivate yourself—it's really up to you (**Figure 10–7**).

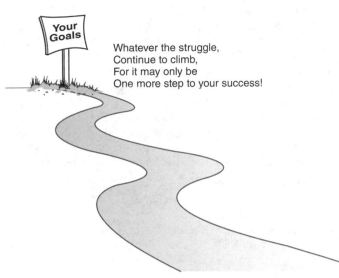

FIGURE 10–7 The road to career success.

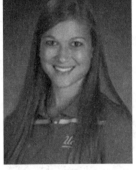

Profile of a Professional

Beth Miller, MS, RD

Director of Performance Nutrition
University of California, Los Angeles Intercollegiate Athletics, Los Angeles, California

Education:
BS in Food, Nutrition, and Dietetics from Tennessee Technological University, Cookeville, Tennessee
MS in Exercise Physiology/Sports Nutrition, Florida State University, Tallahassee, Florida

How did you first hear about dietetics and decide to become a Registered Dietitian?

When I was a freshman in high school, my physician referred me to a see a Registered Dietitian (RD) for a persistent clinical condition that I was dealing with at the time. My visits with the RD had a major impact on my health status and were a vital piece to the puzzle that eventually cleared me of the condition. This interaction with the RD was my first introduction to the profession, and due to the success that I saw firshand, I became very intrigued with dietetics and how important nutrition is to overall health. During my junior year of high school, I had the opportunity to job shadow the same dietitian and complete a report about the field. Ever since, I knew I wanted to become an RD. At this point, however, I just did not know which area of dietetics I wanted to pursue.

What was your route to registration?

I completed the combined Master of Science–Dietetic Internship program at Florida State University.

Where did you complete your supervised practice experience?

My supervised practice experiences were all coordinated through my Dietetic Internship program at Florida State University. For the Community Nutrition experiences, I spent time at various facilities around Tallahassee, Florida, including the American Diabetes Summer Camp for children with type 1 diabetes, Tallahassee Elder Care Services, and the Women, Infants, and Children (WIC) program within the local health department. My Clinical and Foodservice Management rotations were completed at

Harris Methodist Hospital in Fort Worth, Texas. Also, because my internship program had a sports nutrition emphasis, 4 months of my practice experience were spent working in the Florida State Athletic Department.

How have you been involved professionally?

I am a professional member of the Collegiate and Professional Sports Dietitian Association (CPSDA), the Academy of Nutrition and Dietetics, Sports Cardiovascular and Wellness Nutrition DPG, and the American College of Sports Medicine. While a master's student, I served as the Student Co-Chair on the CPSDA board for 2 years. Through this leadership role, I provided guidance for students within the organization as well as organized, edited, and published the student newsletter.

What honors or awards have you received?

- CPSDA and EAS Academy Graduate Scholarship
- Roettger Distinguished Research Award
- Academy of Nutrition and Dietetics Dietetic Intern Scholarship
- NCAA CoSIDA Academic All District Team (Division 1 Cross Country and Track Athlete)
- W.A. Howard Award for 4.0 GPA
- Tennessee Tech University Dean's List and Athletic Director's Honor Roll for eight consecutive semesters

Briefly describe your career path in dietetics. What are you doing now?

I received my first taste of sports nutrition experience during my undergraduate career when I volunteered for the University of Tennessee's Sports Nutrition Department. After this experience, I worked with a private practice dietitian based in Plano, Texas. This position allowed me to work with the Dallas Stars professional hockey team, as well as participate in nutrition blog and social media writing. My next stop on the career path was serving as a Graduate Dietetic Intern for Florida State University (FSU) Performance Nutrition. While at FSU, I worked with all intercollegiate athletic teams, with my primary assignments being football and basketball. After spending 2 years at Florida State, I moved to California for my current position, the Director of Performance Nutrition at University of California, Los Angeles (UCLA).

What excites you about dietetics and the future of our profession?

Nutrition is a fast-paced, ever-changing science. This fact makes our career as dietetics professionals challenging, yet exciting because there is always something new to learn. Advancements in the science, especially in athletic performance and sports nutrition, make our role as sports dietitians even more vital to the success of athletes competing at all levels. More athletes, coaches, and athletic program directors are continuing to realize that sports RDs are dynamic assets to the success of programs in the college, Olympic, professional, and tactical athletic settings. In response to this increased awareness of the science, the National Collegiate Athletic Association (NCAA) deregulated the feeding restrictions of student-athletes in the college setting, opening endless doors for our profession. Our field has grown exponentially in such a short period of time, with new jobs opening up every month. It excites me every day that I am a part of such a thriving field full of energetic professionals.

How is teamwork important to you in your position? How have you been involved in team projects?

In order to ensure the best quality care for the athletes, it is vital that I work hand-in-hand with the multidisciplinary medical team. In a collegiate athletic setting, this team is composed of the team athletic trainers, physicians, psychologists, and athletic performance/strength and conditioning coaches. We all contribute different pieces to the growth and development of the athlete, and it is 100% necessary that we are all on the same page. I interact daily with our athletic trainers and on an as-needed basis with our physicians. Once a month, we have the chance to meet as a full team in our Athlete Care Committee meetings. This meeting provides us a time to discuss high-risk athletes and take a team approach to helping these athletes reach optimal health.

What words of wisdom do you have for future dietetics professionals?
Keep an open mind and gain as many experiences as possible during your educational years. Nutrition is a large field with several practice areas. Find the area you are most passionate about and strive to be the best you can be. This field will continue to thrive as long as we continue to add dedicated, passionate professionals.

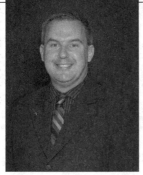

Courtesy of Kevin L. Grzeskowiak

Profile of a Professional

Kevin L. Grzeskowiak, DTR, FMP

Campus General Manager
Unidine Corporation, Deltona, FL

Education:
AS in Dietetic Technician, Madison Area Technical College, Madison, Wisconsin

How did you first hear about dietetics and decide to become a Dietetic Technician, Registered (DTR)?
It all started when I was in high school working as a dietary assistant at a long-term care facility. I wanted to take our Dining Services department to the next level, so I was introduced to the Certified Dietary Manager (CDM) program. However, I felt that the abilities of the CDM were limited so I sought out a Registered Dietitian (RD) program. This program, I felt, was too focused on clinical nutrition. Finally I found the DTR program so I could have the best of both worlds (clinical and foodservice). As a DTR, I could provide expert food systems management to bring services to the next level while having the clinical knowledge to effectively support the RD.

In what types of facilities did you gain your supervised practice experience?
There were a variety of facilities where I gained practice experience. During my management rotation, I was at Lodi Good Samaritan Center in Lodi, Wisconsin. I conducted in-service employee education, long-term care clinical charting, menu planning, purchasing, and procurement. During my clinical rotation, I was at Divine Savior Hospital in Portage, Wisconsin. I conducted discharge diet instruction, acute care patient charting, meal rounds, and department meetings. I also had supervised experience in WIC clinics in Wisconsin and school food systems management. My management practicum was at Attic Angel Place in Middleton, Wisconsin, where I participated in the planning of their new kitchen and dining operation.

Do you have any advanced degree(s)?
I do not have any advanced degrees because the DTR credential has already served me well in preparing me for my advanced career in supporting multiple facilities and varieties of services. I did take the Foodservice Management Professional exam from the National Restaurant Association to earn the credential FMP, so I am diversified as a restaurant manager as well. I also am a registered ServSafe Instructor and Examination Proctor.

How are you involved professionally?
I was elected a Commissioner with the Commission on Dietetic Registration (CDR) of the Academy of Nutrition and Dietetics. I am also a member of the Competency Assurance Panel with CDR, and member of the DTR Exam Panel and item writing.

What honors or awards have you received?
- 5 Star Regional Account for Prescott Valley Samaritan Center
- Regional Account of the Year for Florida Hospital DeLand

• Patient Satisfaction Award for Florida Hospital DeLand
• Retail Excellence Award for Florida Hospital Waterman
• National Account of the Year with Florida Hospital Waterman.

Briefly describe your career path in dietetics. What are you doing now?
I am in management with the role of Director of Dining Departments. This is my passion because this is the area where I feel that I can truly make a difference for the people I serve. I also can give the people I manage the same opportunities I had so they can grow as well. You always want to hold the door open to provide opportunities for the next person after you to pass through. Management also gives you the autonomy to steer your own destiny.

What excites you about dietetics and the future of our profession?
For the DTR, being diversified in both management and clinical operations makes so many opportunities possible. It is so important that the RD has the management and clinical knowledge and support of the DTR to effectively and efficiently direct food and nutrition systems of operation.

How is teamwork important to you in your position? How have you been involved in team projects?
Teamwork is essential to effective operations. No one person has all the answers, and when multiple disciplines have their stake in operations, it makes the entire operation grow. Team projects in which I have been involved include planning and building new foodservice operations, opening new accounts, quality improvement, and labor management.

What words of wisdom do you have for future dietetics professionals?
You need to sell yourself and not wait for others to do it for you. As a DTR, you are an expert in food systems management and a practitioner of nutrition care. No other credential can make this claim. Don't be afraid to fail. If you don't try to advance yourself, you will never know your true potential and power of the DTR. The DTR is the only credential that can effectively and efficiently support the expert nutrition care of the RD in foodservice.

Suggested Activities

1. Begin to research supervised practice program opportunities. What characteristics of a program are important to you (e.g., location, graduate credits, opportunity to specialize, number of interns accepted in each class, cost, length of program)? Visit the Academy of Nutrition and Dietetics website at http://www.eatrightacend.org/ACEND /content.aspx?id=6442485424. Choose at least five internship programs or NDTR programs and visit their websites. Compare the programs with your preferences.

2. Want to learn more success strategies? Go to http://wolfrinke.com /MIWLNEWSLETTER/miwl17-3.htmland read through the article "How to Conquer Stress and Balance Your Life." What strategies would you be willing to incorporate into your life at school and work? What ideas are new to you? How might you adapt them for your own use?

3. More good advice is available at www.rgba.com/article_career_ success.htm. Read the short article on career success strategies. What new strategy did you learn about that you might be willing to try?

4. What's the job market like? Go to www.monster.com. Search for the keyword "dietitian" or "dietetic technician"; in the location box, enter your state. How many positions were listed? Choose one of the positions that you might be interested in sometime in the future. Click the position to find out more about it.

5. The ability to network is important throughout a professional career. Visit https://www.career.Berkeley.edu and search "networking tips." Read the short article on the art of networking. At www.mindtools.com, search for "listening" and watch the short video on listening skills. This is a good reminder of the importance of active listening for good communication.

6. Visit your school's library to determine which nutrition periodicals are available. Carefully examine at least one issue of each, and write one or two sentences describing the journal. For example, one publication might be described as a monthly publication with literature reviews of nutrition research and occasional book reviews. Frequently, many articles in an issue are related to the same topic.

7. Carefully examine an issue of a popular magazine that contains articles on nutrition, such as *Shape* or *Prevention.* Briefly evaluate the reliability and validity of the nutrition content.

8. Attend a continuing education program sponsored by a local dietetic association. Write a report describing what is required of attendees to obtain continuing education credit.

9. Discuss the following scenario: A private-practice dietitian regularly recommends that clients take megadoses of several vitamins. The dietitian bases the recommendation on years of research by a scientist who has testimonial evidence that the treatment works for a number of medical conditions. The dietitian's clients claim to have been helped when traditional medicine has failed. Has the Code of Ethics been violated? What are the issues here?

10. As a follow-up to Activity 9, go to www.eatrightpro.org, scroll to the bottom of the page, and click on the CDR link. At the CDR page, click on "Resources. "Under the "Resources" heading, click the "2009 Code of Ethics" journal article. Read at least the first page of this article. Based on this information, would you change the answer that you gave for Activity 9?

Selected Websites

- http://careerplanning.about.com—Career planning resources at About. com.
- www.CoachWooden.com—Pyramid of Success developed by John Wooden.

Suggested Readings

Abraham J. *Getting Everything You Can Out of All You've Got.* New York: St. Martin's Press; 2000.

Biesemeier C, Marino L, Schofield MK, eds. *Connective Leadership*. Chicago: American Dietetic Association; 2000.

Brandon N. *Self-Esteem at Work*. San Francisco: Jossey-Bass; 1998.

Cherniss C. Emotional intelligence: What it is and why it matters. Consortium for Research on Emotional Intelligence in Organizations website. Available at: http://www.eiconsortium.org/reports/what_is_emotional _intelligence.html. Accessed February 19, 2013.

Drucker P. Managing oneself. *Harvard Business Rev*. 1999;77(2):64–74.

Goleman D. Primal leadership: the hidden driver of great performance. *Harvard Business Rev*. 2001;79(11):42–51.

Johns Hopkins Career Center for Students. http://www.jhu.edu/careers. Accessed March 29, 2016.

Maillet JO. Dietetics in 2017: what does the future hold? *J Am Diet Assoc*. 2002;102(10):1404–1407.

McKay DR. Why you need a mentor. About.com website. Available at: http:// careerplanning.about.com/od/workplacesurvival/a/mentor.htm. Accessed February 19, 2013.

Moore KK. Criteria for acceptance to preprofessional dietetics programs vs. desired qualities of professionals: an analysis. *J Am Diet Assoc*. 1995;95(1):77–81.

Nutrition: Master of public health. University of North Carolina, Gillings School of Public Health website. Available at: http://www.sph.unc.edu /nutr/degrees/#MasterMPH. Accessed February 19, 2013.

Parks SC. The fractured ant hill: a new architecture for sustaining the future. *J Am Diet Assoc*. 2002;102:33.

Seligman M. *Learned Optimism*. New York: Pocket Books; 1998.

Trifari J. From student to professional: making the transition. *The New Social Worker* [serial online] 1999;6(Winter):1.

References

1. Pauline Schatz, EdD, RD. Email message. February 6, 2004. Reprinted by permission of the Estate of Pauline Schatz.

2. Moores S. Six heads are better than one. *ADA Times* 2003;1(Sept/Oct):1–3.

3. Academy of Nutrition and Dietetics. Center for Professional Development. Available at: http://www.eatrightpro.org. Accessed November 11, 2015.

4. Academy of Nutrition and Dietetics. Standards of Practice and Standards of Professional Performance. Available at: http://www.eatrightpro.org. Accessed November 11, 2015.

5. Academy of Nutrition and Dietetics/Commission on Dietetic Registration. Code of Ethics for the Profession of Dietetics. *J Am Diet Assoc*. 1999;99(1):109–113. Also available at: http://www.eatrightpro.org. Accessed November 11, 2015.

6. Drucker P. *Managing the Nonprofit Organization.* New York: HarperCollins; 1990.

7. Wooden J. Wooden on leadership. Available at: http://www.CoachWooden.com. Accessed March 15, 2010.

8. Rinke WJ. Positive Attitude: The Key to Success in Nutrition and Dietetics. Presentation at the Food and Nutrition Conference and Expo, San Antonio, TX, October 26, 2003.

9. Rinke WJ. *The 6 Success Strategies for Winning at Life, Love and Business.* Deerfield Beach, FL: Health Communications; 1996.

10. Rinke WJ. *Positive Attitude: The Key to Peak Performance.* Clarksville, MD: Wolf Rinke Associates; 2003. Available at: http://www.WolfRinke.com/cecredits.html. Accessed February 15, 2004.

Commonly Used Acronyms in the Dietetics Profession

The Academy	Academy of Nutrition and Dietetics
ACEND	Accreditation Council for Education in Nutrition and Dietetics
ANDF	Academy of Nutrition and Dietetics Foundation
ANDPAC	Academy of Nutrition and Dietetics Political Action Committee
ANFP	Association of Nutrition & Foodservice Professionals
AP4	Approved Pre-Professional Practice Program
APC	Academy Position Committee
ASPA	Association of Specialized and Professional Accreditors
ASPEN	American Society of Parenteral and Enteral Nutrition
BHN	Behavioral Health Nutrition (DPG)
BOD	Board of Directors
CADN	Chinese Americans in Dietetics and Nutrition (MIG)
CCN	Certified Clinical Nutritionist
CDE	Certified Diabetes Educator
CD-HCF	Consultant Dietitians in Health Care Facilities (DPG)
CDM, CFPP	Certified Dietary Manager, Certified Food Protection Professional (these two are always used together)
CDR	Commission on Dietetic Registration
CEO	Chief Executive Officer
CFSP	Certified Foodservice Professional
CHES	Certified Health Education Specialist
CNA	Certified Nursing Assistant
CNM	Clinical Nutritional Management (DPG)
CNS	Certified Nutrition Specialist
CNSC	Certified Nutrition Support Clinician
CNSD	Certified Nutrition Support Dietitian
CORPA	Commission on Recognition of Postsecondary Accreditation
CP	Coordinated Program (in Dietetics)
CPE	Continuing Professional Education
CPEU	Continuing Professional Education Units
CPI	Council on Profession Issues
CSG	Board Certified Specialist in Gerontological Nutrition
CSO	Board Certified Specialist in Oncology Nutrition
CSP	Board Certified Specialist in Pediatric Nutrition
CSR	Board Certified Specialist in Renal Nutrition
CSSD	Board Certified Specialist in Sports Dietetics
DBC	Dietitians in Business and Communications (DPG)
DC	Doctor of Chiropractic
DCE	Diabetes Care and Education (DPG)

DDPD	Dietetics in Developmental and Psychiatric Disorders (DPG)
DGCP	Dietitians in General Clinical Practice (DPG)
DHCC	Dietetics in Health Care Communities (DPG)
DI	Dietetic Internship
DICAS	Dietetic Internship Centralized Application System
DM	Dietary Manager
DNS	Dietitians in Nutrition Support (DPG)
DO	Doctor of Osteopathy
DPD	Didactic Program in Dietetics
DPG	Dietetic Practice Group
DPM&R	Dietetics in Physical Medicine and Rehabilitation (DPG)
DT	Dietetic Technician
DTP	Dietetic Technicians in Practice (DPG)
DTR	Dietetic Technician, Registered
EAC	Exhibitor Advisory Council
EFNEP	Expanded Food and Nutrition Education Program
EML	Electronic Mailing List
FADA	Fellow of the American Dietetic Association
FADAN	Filipino American Dietitians and Nutritionists (MIG)
FAND	Fellow of the Academy of Nutrition and Dietetics
FCP	Food and Culinary Professionals (DPG)
FNCE	Food and Nutrition Conference and Exhibition
FPND	Fifty Plus in Nutrition and Dietetics (MIG)
GN	Gerontological Nutritionists (DPG)
GRL	Grassroots Liaison
HA	Health Aging (DPG)
HEC	House Executive Committee
HEN	Hunger and Environmental Nutrition (DPG)
HLT	HOD Leadership Team
HMO	Health Maintenance Organization
HOD	House of Delegates
IDN	Infectious Diseases Nutrition (DPG)
ISPPs	Individualized Supervised Practice Pathways
JAND	*Journal of the Academy of Nutrition and Dietetics*
LD	Licensed Dietitian
LDN	Licensed Dietitian/Nutritionist
LHDN	Latinos and Hispanics in Dietetics and Nutrition (MIG)
LL	Legislative Leader
LNC	Legislative Network Coordinator
LPN	Licensed Practical Nurse
LVN	Licensed Vocational Nurse
MCO	Managed Care Organization
MD	Medical Doctor
MDN	Muslims in Dietetics and Nutrition (MIG)
MFNS	Management in Food and Nutrition Systems (DPG)
MIG	Member Interest Group
MNPG	Medical Nutrition Practice Group (DPG)
MSW	Master's Degree in Social Work
MVC	Member Value Committee
NCC	Nutrition in Complementary Care (DPG)
NCP	Nutrition Care Process
NDEP	Nutrition and Dietetic Educators and Preceptors
NE	Nutrition Entrepreneurs (DPG)
NEHP	Nutrition Educators of Health Professionals (DPG)
NEP	Nutrition Education for the Public (DPG)
NET/NETP	Nutrition Education and Training Program

NNM	National Nutrition Month
NNN	Nationwide Nutrition Network
NOBDN	National Organization of Blacks in Dietetics and Nutrition (MIG)
NOMN	National Organization of Men in Nutrition (MIG)
NSI	Nutrition Screening Initiative
NSPS	Nutrition Services Payment Systems
OA	Overeaters Anonymous
ODY	Outstanding Dietitian of the Year
ON DPG	Oncology Nutrition (DPG)
OT	Occupational Therapist/Therapy
PA	Physician Assistant
PHCN	Public Health/Community Nutrition (DPG)
PID	Professional Issues Delegates
PNPG	Pediatric Nutrition (DPG)
POW	Program of Work
PT	Physical Therapist/Therapy
QM	Quality Management
RD	Registered Dietitian
RDN	Registered Dietitian Nutritionist
RDPG	Renal Dietitians (DPG)
RDTY	Recognized Dietetic Technician of the Year
RN	Registered Nurse
RNP	Registered Nurse Practitioner
RPG	Research (DPG)
RYDY	Recognized Young Dietitian of the Year
SAC	State Associations Committee
SCAN	Sports, Cardiovascular, and Wellness Nutritionists (DPG)
SDA	Student Dietetic Association
SFNS	School Foodservice and Nutrition Specialist
SGA	State Government Affairs
SNE	Society of Nutrition Education
SNS	School Nutrition Services (DPG)
SOE	Standards of Education
SOPP	Standards of Professional Practice
TOPS	Take Off Pounds Sensibly
TJC	The Joint Commission
USDA	United States Department of Agriculture
USDE	United States Department of Education
VN	Vegetarian Nutrition (DPG)
WIC	Women, Infants, and Children
WH	Women's Health (DPG)
WM	Weight Management (DPG)

Index